"Death Is a
Living Process"

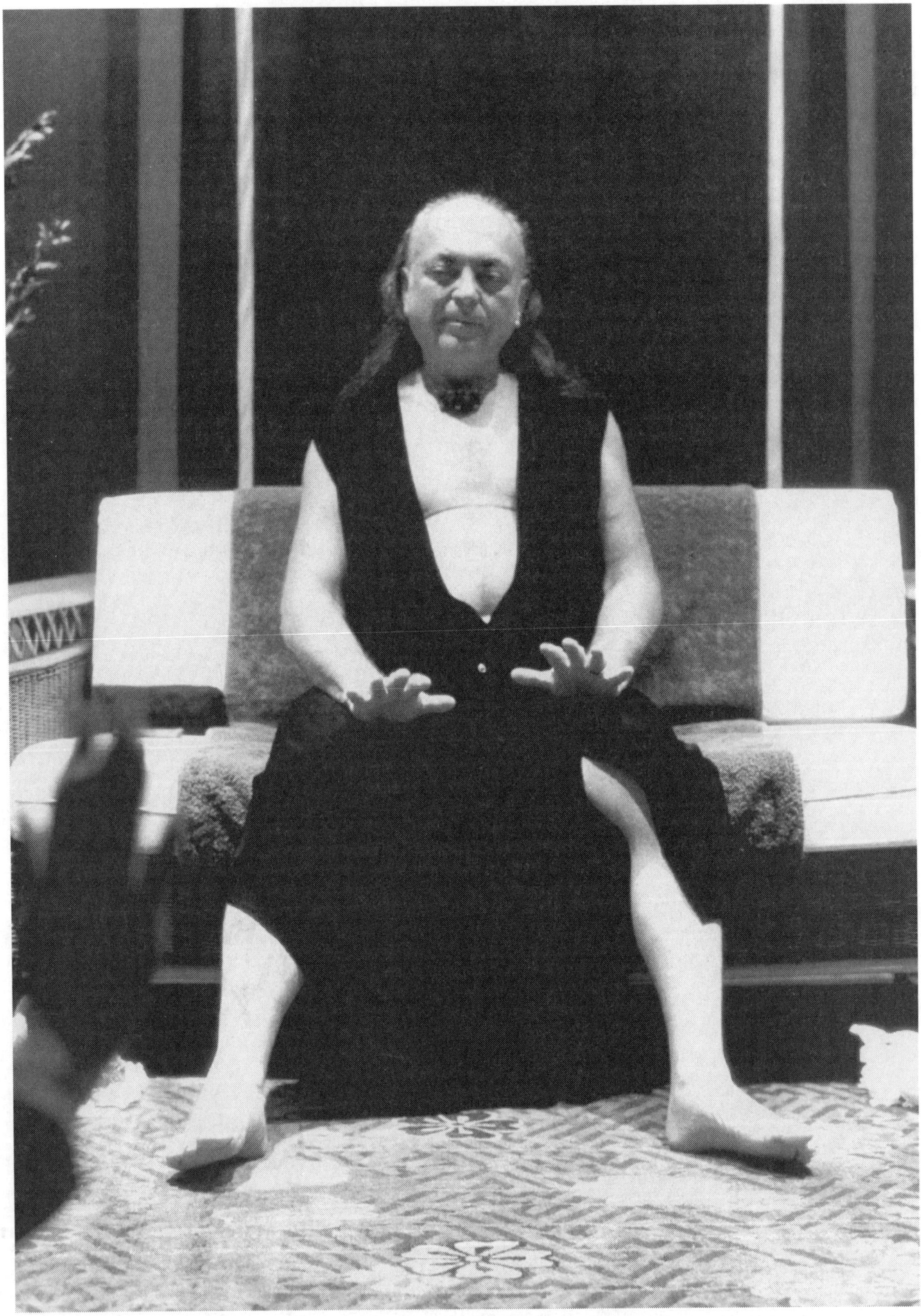

The Divine World-Teacher,
Ruchira Avatar Adi Da Samraj

"Death Is a Living Process"

The Mate Moce Guide to Serving the Dying

A Practical Resource for Practitioners of the Way of Adidam
Based on the Wisdom-Teaching of
The Divine World-Teacher,
Ruchira Avatar Adi Da Samraj

Prepared by the Staff of Mate Moce,
the Death and Dying Ministry of
the Eleutherian Pan-Communion of Adidam

THE DAWN HORSE PRESS
MIDDLETOWN, CALIFORNIA

NOTE TO THE READER

All who study the Way of Adidam or take up its practice should remember that they are responding to a Call to become responsible for themselves. They should understand that they, not Avatar Adi Da Samraj or others, are responsible for any decision they make or action they take in the course of their lives of study or practice.

The devotional, Spiritual, functional, practical, relational, cultural, and formal community practices and disciplines referred to in this book are appropriate and natural practices that are voluntarily and progressively adopted by members of the four congregations of Adidam (as applicable for each of the congregations and as appropriate to the personal circumstance of each individual). Although anyone may find these practices useful and beneficial, they are not presented as advice or recommendations to the general reader or to anyone who is not a member of one of the four congregations of Adidam. And nothing in this book is intended as a diagnosis, prescription, or recommended treatment or cure for any specific "problem", whether medical, emotional, psychological, social, or Spiritual. One should apply a particular program of treatment, prevention, cure, or general health only in consultation with a licensed physician or other qualified professional.

"Death Is a Living Process" is formally authorized for publication by the Ruchira Sannyasin Order of the Tantric Renunciates of Adidam, for distribution to formally acknowledged devotees of the Divine World-Teacher, Ruchira Avatar Adi Da Samraj, and to members of the public who may be moved to respond to *"Death Is a Living Process"* (The Ruchira Sannyasin Order of the Tantric Renunciates of Adidam is the senior Spiritual and Cultural Authority within the formal gathering of formally acknowledged devotees of the Divine World-Teacher, Ruchira Avatar Adi Da Samraj.)

Cover photograph by Cliff Baker

ISBN 1-57097-085-8

Printed in the United States of America

Produced by the Ruchirasala of Adidam
in cooperation with the Dawn Horse Press,
a division of the Eleutherian Pan-Communion of Adidam

CONTENTS

About the Mate Moce Ministry

The Divine World-Teacher, Ruchira Avatar Adi Da Samraj has indicated that it is useful for practitioners of the Way of Adidam to serve other devotees at the time of their death, in order to create an appropriate and auspicious circumstance for the death transition.

At the present time, particularly in the Western world, those who are dying are commonly served by outside professionals rather than in the context of an intimate sacred gathering. Thus, in order to respond to Avatar Adi Da's Instructions in this regard, and to bring intimate and loving support to each other in the death process, a group of devotees of Avatar Adi Da came together in 1982 to form a death and dying ministry informed by His Divine Wisdom and practical Instruction. In 1983, Avatar Adi Da Samraj Blessed this ministry with the name "Mate Moce" (pronounced MAH-tay MO-thay), a name with an unusual history.

On a tour of Naitauba Island (now also known as Adidam Samrajashram) when Adi Da Samraj first arrived there, He heard of a woman named Mate Moce, who had lived on the island some years earlier. She had been named in this way: Shortly before she was born, a resident in her village had died in sleep, and so the new baby was given the name Mate (death) Moce (sleep), in keeping with the Fijian custom of naming the newborn babies after noteworthy events occurring around the time of their birth. Dying in one's sleep implies to Fijians a peaceful death. Thus "Mate Moce" is the Fijian equivalent of "Easy Death".

Presently, Mate Moce, the death and dying ministry of the community of Adidam, serves practitioners of the Way of Adidam who are dying, and their intimates, in the following ways:

■ By providing direct help with and service to the death of formal practitioners of the Way of Adidam, including the practical management of the three-day vigil that follows the death of a practitioner, the right orientation of those who serve this occasion, and the compassionate, formal guidance of the entire circumstance surrounding a death.

■ By providing general counseling to practitioners of the Way of Adidam in all matters related to death and dying.

■ By offering educational materials, courses, and audiotapes for members of the four congregations of Adidam on the right understanding of death and dying, as Revealed and Given by Avatar Adi Da.

■ By developing educational materials and seminars for the public about understanding death from the point of view of the Way of Adidam.

Introduction

The Western world is a death-denying society. Every day people die in secluded hospital rooms surrounded by technology rather than by the people who love them. Bodies are whisked off to the morgue and from there to the funeral home, where they are embalmed and perfumed and made to look as though only sleeping—called the "memory image" in the funeral industry. Family and friends are left out of the entire process.

While institutions like hospice are attempting to make the death process more humane, Avatar Adi Da Samraj has Given Instruction to His devotees which goes far beyond mere benevolent service. The practice of serving the dead or dying in the Way of Adidam is Spiritually profound and ecstatic. The experience of participating in a vigil in the Way of Adidam, with its complete focus on Invocation of Avatar Adi Da and surrender into His Divine Being, greatly serves those performing the vigil as well as the one who has died. By Adi Da's Divine Grace, even the grieving process is significantly shortened.

◆ ◆ ◆

In this Guide, you will find detailed instructions on serving the death transition. Part One includes recommendations relative to preparing for death (your own or someone else's). Part Two has information about serving the death process itself—for both practitioners of Adidam and their loved ones who are not practitioners of Adidam. Part Three focuses on instructions relative to performing a three-day vigil, including practical advice on how to preserve the body. Inspiring Leelas in Part Four illustrate how these unique forms of service have been done in Adidam and how Avatar Adi Da Samraj has Guided His devotees in their death transition. Part Five is specifically about the death of children and helping children to understand the death of others. Part Six includes readings that will serve your understanding of Avatar Adi Da's Wisdom-Teaching on the death process.

Part Seven, at the end of this Guide, includes the necessary legal form that all devotees must complete in order to have their death transition served as smoothly as possible.

Yellow "Alert Cards" can be obtained from your local CSM or Mate Moce representative. Devotees should carry a yellow alert card with them at all times, to prevent autopsy, embalming, or organ donation, and to give the care provider emergency phone numbers to call.

Please note that publications recommended in this manual that are not based on Adidam need to be read with discrimination in the light of Ruchira Avatar Adi Da Samraj's Instructions on the death and dying process.

May this guide help all practitioners of Adidam to a deeper surrender in love and Happiness to Avatar Adi Da Samraj.

PART ONE

Preparing for the Death Transition

Part One of the guide is an overview of practicalities associated with the preparation for death. Avatar Adi Da's book *Easy Death* should be studied extensively, along with associated coursework, to gain an understanding of the psychological and Spiritual preparation for the death transition. This section is only intended to summarize such study and point out practical considerations for all members of Adidam and especially for the terminally ill.

Death Is a Necessary Process

A Talk by Ruchira Avatar Adi Da Samraj

AVATAR ADI DA SAMRAJ: Fear of death is anxiety, or emotional recoil, experienced in anticipation of the event. Such advance fear is basically the result of a failure to observe the death process in others and to study the death process through systematic education and self-observation.

Death is a necessary, purposeful, and ultimately benign psycho-physical process. It is similar to the process of giving birth, except that it occurs to both males and females. You must study the death process bodily and through observing others. Above all, tension and fear must be relaxed during the death process (as it must be by a woman in childbirth). You must relax and release, as when going to sleep, in a feeling of deep trust, love, and surrender to the Divine Reality on Which the process depends. What is on the "other side" of the death process may or may not be revealed to you beforehand, but it will certainly be revealed to you when it actually happens! Therefore, your only responsibility is to study, prepare for, and rightly engage the death process itself, much as a woman approaching childbirth. In the birth process, the newly born enters this world via the lower bodily organs of the mother. In the death process, the living being enters a new world via the crown of the head of the dying body (which, in effect, is the "mother" of the living being). You must learn how to cooperate with the death process as a natural event leading to this end.

The failure of such cooperation tends to make the death process painful and disturbing, even as the birth process can be for the mother who fails to surrender and cooperate with the event. And if you do not surrender with attention, feeling, breath, and body in cooperation with the death process, you will tend to interfere with the ultimate event of release and separation from this body and world—which, like sleep, is intended to refresh and strengthen the phenomenal being in preparation for a rebirth, or resumed embodiment. Resistance during the actual death process makes the necessary transition difficult, and you may thereby force yourself into a pattern of psychic withholding whereby you remain fixed in a ritual of illusory and frustrated association with past experiential aspects of the now dying or receding body and world. (In that case, attention does not pass freely to the crown of the head and beyond, but it becomes locked in dreamlike associations with memories, vital associations, and various aspects of experience in this passing body and world.)

You should prepare for death as a process of complete surrender and release of all physical, emotional, and mental clinging to the present body-mind, its relations, and this world. Your death should be a complete release of this present "school" and a complete abandonment of the present design and content of your conditional self. You should fully consent to die at the moment of death, and so be released toward what is new and awaiting you above and beyond the "realities" of the present body-mind. Your ability to do this will be either enhanced or limited to the same degree you are able to surrender while alive in the Divine Love-Bliss-Consciousness That Is Real God. Therefore, in order for death to be an ecstatic transition for you, you must not only study and prepare for the specific and terminal process of death itself, but while alive you must also devote yourself to an ecstatic or ego-transcending way of life. [*Easy Death*, pp. 52-53]

Basic Recommendations from Avatar Adi Da Regarding Death

The following four points summarize Avatar Adi Da's basic recommendations about the death transition. These points are important for all members of Adidam to know and take appropriate action. Items one and two involve preparation of legal documents previous to terminal illness and death and will be discussed in the following pages. Items three and four, relating to care of the body after the death transition, will be discussed in Parts Two and Three of this Guide.

1. Extraordinary, life-prolonging measures are discouraged in someone who is terminally ill.

2. The body should be as undisturbed as possible for three days after death. If possible, there should be no embalming, organ donation, or autopsy. Even a bowel puncture, often performed in hospitals right after death, is to be discouraged.

3. A vigil should be held for three days to serve the release of the one who has died.

4. After three days, the body should be cremated. This further serves the release of attachment to the body as there is no more body to be attached to. Ashes should then be scattered, preferably in the ocean.

Preparations All Practitioners of Adidam Should Make to Provide Legal Protection

The medical establishment has become very skilled in keeping individuals alive long after they would have died naturally, and often people are kept alive in nothing more than an unresponsive vegetative state. Avatar Adi Da has Said the following about this practice:

The vulgarization of human life is something that must be changed, and among the things that must be changed is the kind of treatment the dead generally receive, even the kind of treatment the sick receive from medical people whose sole purpose is to keep the individual alive. Only on some level is that purpose laudable and right. As long as life can be maintained, as long as the individual can exist fruitfully and consciously, it is appropriate enough to take life-saving measures. But much of what is being done has the purpose not to provide a vehicle of embodiment for someone's Spiritual practice but rather to fulfill the vulgar idealism of keeping someone alive, which is based on fear and non-sensitivity to the state of someone who is dying. [Easy Death, *p. 274*]

To ensure the appropriate medical and legal protection for those who are terminally ill or seriously injured, all devotees are encouraged to complete a Durable Power of Attorney for Health Care or its equivalent where they live.

The Durable Power of Attorney for Health Care (DPAHC) is similar to a Living Will, which instructs one's doctor and family to refrain from measures to prolong the process of dying when one is terminally ill and unable to communicate one's wishes (as in a coma). But the DPAHC is more useful because it also names people to make health care decisions for you if you are unable to do so. Devotees should make a copy of their DPAHC to be kept by their Radiant Life Clinic or Mate Moce representative and keep the original with their important papers. If you are facing a medical procedure which could potentially become life-threatening, you should have a copy of your DPAHC introduced into your hospital chart.

The DPAHC is obviously important when a person is in a coma and cannot make health care decisions for himself or herself, but it is also important if someone's mental functioning is impaired in other ways. A number of devotees have had mental functioning impaired by brain cancer or dementia, and the persons named in their DPAHCs (the attorneys-in-fact) had many and varied decisions to make.

The DPAHC is also useful after death has occurred. A hospital will not release a body, even to a funeral director, without an authorized signature. The signature could be that of a spouse or family member or a person named in the DPAHC. In Adidam, many couples are not legally married and family members are often many miles away—in addition to usually being non-devotees who might choose to have the body handled differently than a practitioner of Adidam might. So, once again, it is very important to have this document.

The DPAHC can also be of value when it comes time to cremate. In California, the DPAHC includes instructions about cremation, but this is not so in other states. If you are using a

DPAHC which is legal in a state where cremation is not included in the DPAHC, in consultation with a legal professional, the following wording could be added:

> "My agent is to handle the disposition of my remains. I also give my health care agent the right to transfer, transport, and make any arrangements for my body after death which my health care agent deems necessary or consistent in his sole judgement with my wishes as expressed in this document."

Funeral directors are wary of cremating without proper consent. Without a DPAHC or without a family member's consent, they would probably not cremate the body. This is yet one more reason to handle your legal forms so as to prevent all these potential complications.

Note that the people you name in your DPAHC to make health care decisions should preferably be devotees who live close by. If you move, then do another form. Decisions and signatures are hard to get long distance.

The DPAHC written for devotees—and legal in the state of California—is in Part Seven of this guide. Every devotee should research what is legal in their own state, province, or country. As mentioned above, extra wording could be added to account for cremation instructions if necessary.

In the past, devotees also completed a form called "Funeral Directions", but that is no longer required since everything of legal significance is covered in the DPAHC or can be added with the above wording.

Devotees should also fill out a yellow Alert Card (which can be obtained from your local CSM or Mate Moce representative). This is to be carried with you at all times, close to your driver's license. It gives brief instructions and phone numbers to call for someone who might find you seriously injured or dead, so that you can be properly served.

It is important to inform people you name as your attorneys-in-fact on your DPAHC, as this is a big responsibility. Talk with your family members about how you wish to be treated when you are dying and after death. This will help greatly in reducing conflict, which is so common in families when someone dies.

Renunciation in Preparation for Death

AVATAR ADI DA SAMRAJ: The Divine Spirit is not afraid of death. Therefore, if you Commune with the Divine Spirit, if you are really intimate with the Divine Spirit in this present moment, then the body-mind's reactivity to death relaxes. The more profoundly you enter into heart-Communion with Me, the less you associate with the tendencies of the body-mind. Death can be easy in that case. If you are entered into the Divine Spirit in the process of death, then the body will go through the natural process of death without aberrating your consciousness. Death will be natural, easy surrender. There will be no clinging and no fear.

Death should be, and in general can be, easy, natural in this sense. But if death is to be easy, you must be linked to the Divine Reality That Transcends the body-mind. Otherwise, if you are simply identified with the body-mind and contracting, you are, as a matter of course, going to awaken in fear at the point of dying, and you are going to awaken in many other emotions and reactions that will determine your destiny after death. [*Easy Death*, p. 105]

It is very important that each one of us consciously prepare for death, both practically and Spiritually, so that, when we are actively dying, we will be able to engage the process fully. The entire practice of the Way of Adidam serves to prepare us to let go of all attachments to body, mind, and world.

In *Easy Death*, Avatar Adi Da says:

Your consciousness must become one with This Divine Reality. You must magnify your association with That, enter into heart-Communion with That, rather than reinforce the persona, or the egoic tendencies of attention. In this way, you prepare yourself for death, but you also live well. You live in Wisdom. And, if you have lived a lifetime in this Wisdom, then death will certainly become a profound event, not different in kind from profound meditation. [p. 107]

Avatar Adi Da Instructed one devotee who was approaching the death transition to practice "intensely for the sake of purification and release of conditions in anticipation of this transition, instead of being preoccupied with holding on, or animating a merely social disposition". He Said it was a time for this devotee to be practicing in "an exemplary and renunciate manner".

Thus, in preparing for death, avoid engaging the social personality. A practice of maintaining some hours of silence every day is useful. Work toward releasing friends, intimate partner, children, etc. Bind yourself instead to our Beloved Guru Who Says, "I Provide the Means for the 'Bonding' of all beings to Myself, so that they may be Liberated from samsaric outward-directedness by being drawn into the integrity of the body-mind in devotion to Me, and then Beyond even that vehicle into My Divine Domain, via the seventh stage Yoga." [*Free Daist*, 4th Quarter 1994, p. 14]

It is useful to study, in addition to *Easy Death*, the Leelas in Part Four of this guide. They are full of Beloved Adi Da's Blessing Instruction to those of His devotees who were in the death process, particularly on renunciation as preparation for the transition.

Forgive and Be Forgiven

When someone learns he or she have a terminal illness, Beloved Adi Da Says that such a one first needs to settle his or her affairs and then "forgive and be forgiven". The need to forgive and be forgiven is a form of business that must be handled. If it is not, it will cause clinging to the body-mind even as it is clearly dying. People with long unresolved issues and old emotional holdings find it difficult to simply let go.

Avatar Adi Da Samraj Gives us Instruction about forgiveness in the following Talk from 1985.

AVATAR ADI DA SAMRAJ: There are two forms of forgiveness, or two options that you may choose in relation to anyone. The greater option is to grant forgiveness in the form of great energy, love, regard, help, friendship, and upliftment. That is one option, and, in certain relations and in certain moments, it is an option you can call upon yourself to exercise. The other option, which is really the fundamental motive or force of forgiveness, is to ignore the offense, to forget about it, to not give attention to it. Perhaps the fundamental definition of forgiveness is to just forget or ignore the offense. Such forgetting has the force of forgiveness because it gives no negative energy.

You may be troubling yourself because you cannot forgive those who have negative feelings about you, in that you cannot love them and just be happy about them. Perhaps in some moments every now and then you achieve such love, but you are struggling as if forgiveness and right relationship to these individuals means you must magnify radiant love toward them. You need not feel guilty because you cannot do that. If you can do it, fine—to do so is healing and the ultimate form of forgiveness. However, the form of ultimate forgiveness for which you are responsible is forgetting, or ignoring, or non-attention.

Therefore, give no attention to those who want to harm you. Do not give them any attention, and you will, therefore, not give them any negative energy, you will not curse them. Forget about them. Put your attention somewhere else. Put your attention on Me.

Just so with our own difficulties or the difficulties of others with whom you are intimate—if you cannot give radiant, loving, blessing energy, that is all right. It is simply not your moment for such energy. You can ignore difficulties, however. You can forget about the offense, you can not talk about it, you can be reticent, you can be silent, you can occupy yourself with your practice of Invocation of Me. You can do all those things, can you not? Then forget. That <u>is</u> forgiveness.

Forgiveness is to forget, to not make curses, to not hold others to account. You can always do that. Therefore, always do it. Then, in unique moments, grant great energy and attention, full of blessing and support and helpfulness. Do not feel guilty if you cannot. Do it when you are Given My Avataric Divine Grace to do it. But, in all moments, forgive by ignoring and forgetting. Have nothing to do with the offense and go about your own business.

To do this is not a curse. In fact, it is the denial of curses. Therefore, at least forget. You can do that by Invoking Me, feeling Me, breathing Me, and serving Me.

Do the practice of Adidam in general and in relation to the difficult moments of life. Do it with one another. Do not spend time in talking about your "case" or anyone else's. You need not aggravate yourself constantly with the difficulties of others. You have your own difficulties anyway! You know the moments that are your charismatic moments of blessing and helping and touching and laying on of hands. Those moments only occur at certain times, however. Most of the time the difficulties of others are their own business. Fail to curse them by forgetting them. Occupy yourself with devotional Communion with Me and your own real practice. Do not pass on bad thoughts, which are effectively curses. Just forget about it. That is forgiveness. That is how even the forgiveness of God is described traditionally. Real God Forgets. To forget is to forget to curse. To ignore is forgiveness. It is the principal form of forgiveness, and you can be responsible for it.

You need not feel guilt because you cannot bless and love and radiate to everyone who lives or who curses you. Ignore their curses, ignore their faults, ignore their person, and occupy yourself with Real God. Curse no one. Love them or forget them. Do not curse. You need not feel guilt, because you can always forget to curse. Simply put your attention somewhere else, and do not imagine that you are guilty because you have not magnified great blessing. Such blessing is virtue, but it is My special Grace for special moments. Do not curse.

All you need do to not curse is to forget about it and put your attention somewhere else—go to the Communion Hall. Serve Me. Study. Overcome the thought. You can do that. You already know that you can do that, but do it rigorously, constantly, and be sensitive to those moments in which you can magnify great energy, great enthusiasm, great feeling. When the capability for giving special attention to someone arises, give it. Do not fail to do so. You will not be able to help yourself in any case, so magnify your feelings in those moments. To do that is not forgiveness—it is blessing. Forgiveness is to forget about it and go about your business.

Love all your friends. Love all beings. Be liberated from all otherness, which is painful, a form of suffering. Otherness is something to be liberated from entirely. How can you be liberated from otherness? Only through love. Love Me, the Avataric Divine Realizer, the Avataric Divine Revealer, and the Avataric Divine Self-Revelation of Real God. Don't you know? Have you not discovered That? [Crazy Wisdom magazine, Vol. 5, No. 9]

Practical Care for the Terminally Ill

This section covers the practical concerns that affect a person's quality of life when he or she has a terminal illness.

In the first part, we look into home care versus hospital care and suggest ways that home care can be made relatively easy and affordable. We then look into the physical care of the dying person and ways to reduce his or her pain while actually enhancing that person's participation in the death process. We also talk briefly about how to serve someone who is comatose.

Home Care versus Hospital Care

If you can make the choice to manage someone's physical care at home, you will have more control over the circumstance of that person's life and death. You may be able to create a conscious, loving, and supportive environment. Home care of the terminally ill is an increasingly recognized option that many are beginning to choose.

Though the decision to care for your friend or loved one yourself may seem overwhelming to you at first, there is help. Licensed practical nurses and physicians can come to your home and instruct you, and home health aides may be able to provide ongoing care. You may wish to contact a home health agency or hospice organization near your home and discuss ways in which they can assist you. As a formal practitioner of the Way of Adidam, you will also want to discuss this matter with your local Mate Moce and Radiant Life Clinic representative.

The idea of home death is still fairly new to many practicing physicians. So don't be surprised if your loved one's physician is not supportive of the idea, but don't be discouraged either. Marshal your arguments and present them forcefully but with good humor—don't be overbearing, and don't view the physician as an adversary. Persistence in stating your case may be necessary.

Recommended Reading:

A full consideration of home care versus hospital care is given in chapter two of Deborah Duda's book entitled, *Coming Home: A Guide to Dying at Home with Dignity* (New York: Aurora Press, 1987).

Financing of Home Care

In the United States, the costs of home care can sometimes be covered by Medicare, private insurance, or state funded programs. Often a call to your local, licensed home health agency or hospice organization will give you the best information and guidance. There is an increasing trend in the health care field to move terminal patients out of the hospital setting and provide palliative and comfort care in the home, where the dying process will be allowed to proceed in a natural fashion. At home, your loved one is not going to be resuscitated (unless medical teams are called) or placed in the Intensive Care Unit when the death process begins.

Deciding When and Whether to Use Health Care Professionals

There is really no reason to give the full-time care of one another up to the medical profession at this most important time unless there isn't sufficient help or expertise available. Of course, you cannot do it alone. It is possible, though, to manage pain or breathing difficulties, for example, with the proper medication and oxygen equipment; this requires some supervision by a nurse and/or physician, but not the full-time care or hospitalization that is commonly given.

Practitioners of Adidam often have the manpower and expertise—not to mention the disposition and outlook—to provide for each other. If not, it is fine to use outside medical help. If you prudently "shop around", you should be able to find people who will support your wishes and intentions.

You will be far better served if, as a part of your interaction with medical professionals and others in clinical settings, you educate people about Avatar Adi Da's "Point of View" on the death process. Assume no limits. Whatever your circumstance is, simply engage it as your service to Avatar Adi Da Samraj and allow that circumstance to become your given sadhana.

Physical Care

Physical comfort and quality of life are important considerations when trying to manage the symptoms of someone whose body is failing. Often one of the first signs of such failure is increasing weakness. The individual may be unable to stand or walk and may shortly become bedbound. For one who is confined to bed, good skin care is very important to prevent pressure areas from developing into very painful bed sores. Your visiting nurse or home health aide will be able to show you how to manage the safety and comfort of a bedbound individual. Adequate fluid intake is also very important, particularly for someone who has little appetite or cannot swallow easily. If the individual cannot consume solid foods, his or her nutritional requirements could be met by the fluids consumed. Various high protein blender drinks are often recommended for such individuals.

You may see many symptoms of decline—shortness of breath, swelling of the body, fever, nausea, vomiting, and loss of bowel and bladder control. These symptoms can be quite embarrassing to the terminally ill or dying person. Add to that his or her increasing (or even total) dependency on others for such basic functions as feeding, toileting, and mobility, and such an individual may feel that he or she has no dignity or worth. Under such circumstances, it may be very helpful and reassuring to talk with your intimate one about the need for surrender. The opportunity to be close to someone who must receive physical help in this way can be wonderful for you as well as for that person. It can be a time of intimacy and sharing between family members that can truly upgrade the quality of anyone's final days—and, even more importantly, enable the dying person to release concerns and, thus, the hold on this life. Many have reported that this time of caring for an intimate has healed a lifetime of missed communications or past difficulties.

Pain Management

To see someone you love in pain is always very distressing, but there is much that can be done to help make such a person more comfortable. Relaxation exercises, massage, and touch can all serve greatly to reduce anxiety and increase comfort. However, most people who are in continuous physical pain need some kind of chemical relief or else the quality of their hours and days may become unbearable. Avatar Adi Da has not recommended that we avoid pain medication, if it is necessary, and we do not suggest that it be avoided for reasons of pride or ideology.

The principle is to maintain the best possible level of consciousness for the individual, so that he or she is able to engage the death process with as much clarity and ease as possible. For practitioners of the Way of Adidam, we recommend using alternatives to narcotics as much as possible to alleviate pain, so that the level of consciousness is not dulled. Anti-inflammatory drugs may be used to ease some kinds of pain and mild tranquilizers or sedatives may be helpful alternatives to narcotics. Under the influence of narcotics, the dying individual may be less able to distinguish between internal phenomena arising in the death process and less able to follow the direct and upward surrender in feeling-Contemplation of Avatar Adi Da Samraj's Avatarically-Born bodily (human) Divine Form.

Persons in a Coma

People may enter a state of profound unconsciousness for many different reasons and remain in a comatose state for varying lengths of time. Since comatose patients do not respond to stimuli, it is generally believed that they do not receive stimuli. However, this is not true in the case of the hearing function. Comatose people do hear and are often aware of what is going on around them, but they are in an altered state of consciousness similar to a trance state. People often slip into a coma shortly before they die, and it is important to continue to serve and instruct and help them in the process of letting go. Be sensitive to the comatose person you are serving and refrain from talking about him or her where he or she can hear you.

There is a good book on this subject called *Coma: The Dream Body near Death* by Arnold Mindell (Arkana, 1995). He explores various ways of communicating with and helping people who are in comatose states.

PART TWO

Serving the Dying

This part of the guide begins with essential general instruction about the death process and how to serve that in an other. Following are very practical, step-by-step instructions on what to do when someone you know is dying or has died.

How to Serve the Dying Person

A Talk by Ruchira Avatar Adi Da Samraj
May 31, 1980

DEVOTEE: Beloved Adi Da, my mother is dying, and tomorrow I am flying to be with her. I would like to know how to serve her best. She has lost the use of speech and movement, but she responds with feeling to some things around her.

AVATAR ADI DA SAMRAJ: Has she outer awareness?

DEVOTEE: Yes, but she has no mind.

AVATAR ADI DA SAMRAJ: Does she have memory? That is, does she know who people are?

DEVOTEE: No, not really, though she smiles when she hears I am coming to see her.

AVATAR ADI DA SAMRAJ: There is really nothing unusual about her state. She has physical sensation and outer awareness. She responds emotionally. She notices events at some level. Although dying, she is basically there. You can, therefore, relate to her through all the means whereby you would ordinarily relate to her.

Over the years, I have Told many stories of the summer I spent as a chaplain in a mental hospital during My training in a Christian seminary. Among My obligations was to comfort people who were dying or close to death. I remember on one occasion going to see a woman who had no outer awareness whatsoever. To talk to her or to try to elicit her acknowledgment of Me as a human being was futile. Still, I was capable of all My bodily and emotional and mental activities, even though she was not, and, therefore, I could approach her and serve her Spiritually.

Just so, you also have all your faculties and abilities, and you are fully alive as My devotee and conscious in this world. Therefore, you should do for your mother all the things that I recommend and that you know to do in the company of someone who is dying.

You are not yet, at least, limited by your mother's absence of awareness. She still has the basic faculties that make a relationship with her possible. You should speak to her, even if she does not speak to you, and give her the feeling that there is nothing negative between you. If there has been anything negative between you in the past, you should, through your conversation, make it clear to her that you forgive her and that you feel forgiven by her. Make completely clear to her that you no longer feel any limitations in your relationship.

If you like, you can read to her what I have Communicated about the death process and about simply surrendering—that she should have no fear that death will destroy her, that death is simply a transition into other experiences that also pass, that eventually she may resume a human existence, or at least perhaps a personal existence in an environment, and that as she passes through these stages of experience after she leaves this world, she will be given help. It is true that after your death people come to help you, telling you where you are and what is happening to you, just as people do in this realm. Try to bring to her a sense of the reality of her situation, not the dismal downtown expectation that "when you're dead, you're dead", because that view is a completely untrue and worldly and terrible vision.

When the present body becomes too weak to go on, it is quite naturally abandoned, but the process of abandoning the body is not the destruction of the individual being. Light is Indivisible and Indestructible. Light is Eternal and Never-Changing. Because human beings are essentially apparent modifications of Light, they continue to exist after death, but they also continue to undergo transformations. The purpose of your existence is to surrender to Light Itself, until, instead of realizing only the changes and the transformations, you have Realized Perfectly Subjective Light Itself.

Your mother, then, should surrender to Real God, or the One Who is Living her, knowing that Real God is Light and Love and Fullness and Happiness and Purpose and Creative Will, and she should let herself be carried without fear from this world by that Great Influence. Make sure she knows that you love her and that there is nothing unfinished between you and her that demands her attention. Let her feel completely free to relax into the death process when it finally occurs. In the meantime, she should simply surrender, know she is loved, and know that you, as well as the others who are intimate with her and who may also be with her, feel that she loves you. Such heart-felt communications, because they are natural and human, serve the transition at death.

When the event of the death of another finally occurs, although the emotion of sorrow will naturally arise, you should remain My devotee in that moment, and, instead of merely feeling sorrowful, surrender through feeling-Contemplation of Me in that moment, giving the one who has left your company your full permission to release all hold on this present existence. You should release the dying one. You should cooperate with the person's release from this life and not, in effect, try to trap and keep the person here. The process into which he or she is entering arises in Real God and is inevitable. By trusting that process and by continuing to surrender with full feeling and love of Me, you, too, can be adjusted to it.

Thus, you must be active in the event of your mother's death as you are also while she continues to live. You must realize equanimity through your own love and trust of the Divine Process. Then, in the actual event of her death, you must continue to love and trust this Process and give her permission to pass out of her present relationship with you, even to pass completely out of your sight.

In the days following her death, you should allow yourself to be sensitive to any unusual sign of her presence. It is quite typical that, after the death of an intimate, people have dreams or unusual experiences that are synchronous with that person's passage. Such phenomena do not necessarily mean that the person is trying to communicate with you, but simultaneous or associated events typically arise. Therefore, allow yourself to be sensitive, and such events may be part of your own experiential evidence of the realities of this transition that we call "death".

Death is not an ending. Thus, most likely, after a few days those experiences will stop, because the psychic part of the conditional being has separated—not only from the physical body but, in general, from the environment. It has gone on to its further destiny. You may have other experiences from time to time, particularly if you, the person still living, maintain an emotional attachment to the one who has passed.

Generally, however, you should release all of that. Release the person fully as he or she is dying and during the few days after his or her death, until you are yourself completely content and surrendered in devotional Communion with Me and can continue your practice of the Way of Adidam here without lingering in this event.

Avatar Adi Da's Formal Instructions for Dying Practitioners of Adidam

The following are Avatar Adi Da's Instructions to be read to, or by, the dying person. Avatar Adi Da further instructs us that optimally only His Words—and not readings or instructions from other sources—should be used for the transition and vigil of a devotee.

As the individual approaches the death process:

1. "Settle your affairs in this world."

2. "Forgive and be forgiven."

As the individual enters into the death process:

3. "Relax all clinging and attention relative to the relations of your body and mind."

4. "Accept the naturalness, orderliness, and purposiveness of the death process, and relax or surrender into each of its stages as they appear."

5. "Release and relax all fear and simply surrender into cooperation with the death process like a woman in labor—and, like a woman in labor, consciously and bodily accept and feel through even the more painful, embarrassing, unpleasant, or chaotic aspects of the total event."

6. "Outer and bodily awareness will gradually disappear in the death process, but it is not necessary to lose consciousness. Simply keep attention on whatever replaces your present bodily and outer awareness."

7. "As outer awareness begins to subside, begin to practice the 'dead pose'—that is, systematically relax the body beginning at the feet. Relax from the feet progressively toward the crown, withdrawing attention from each lower level to the next."

8. "Continually surrender what arises by keeping attention on the actual and progressive process of death and ultimate emergence from the present body-mind."

9. "Breathe as evenly and easily as possible, but progressively surrender the entire process of sensation, breath, and heartbeat."

10. "Release the body, emotion, and attention into the Divine Life-Current via the central line of the body and toward the crown, until there is emergence from the body-mind via the crown into the next or new dimension of experience."

As the devotee passes out of his or her dying body:

11. "Whatever appearances arise after awareness of the dying body passes, continue to feel through and beyond all recoil of egoic self or toward egoic self—but surrender beyond everything and everyone into the Divine Spiritual Current of My Love-Bliss-Life That Is within and above egoic self and all beings or phenomena."

In Chapter 39 of *The Dawn Horse Testament Of The Ruchira Avatar*, Beloved Adi Da Describes the ascending practice in the Way of Adidam and how to practice with ascended visions. This Instruction may be used with a devotee who has died, as it also describes the ascending process that occurs at death. Be sure to read it slowly, with frequent pauses.

Do Not Hold To any limited object . . . or field . . . that is presently Before You. Do Not Seek To the left or the right. Hold Heart-Feeling and attention To An Upturned View, and Constantly Turn and Yield Toward The Center (Up and Back, Up and Back). Always Feel Beyond what presently appears (or Whatever Is Made Apparent), and Always Be Moved (Up and Back, Up and Back) Toward The Indefinable Central Source-Space Above The Total Crown Of the head.

If I Am Perceived In A (Subtle) Vision Of My Avatarically-Born Bodily (Human) Divine Form, I Will Lead Your attention Upwards. Therefore, If I Appear In (Subtle) Vision—Look Toward Me, Hold On To Me, Ascend With Me. . . . If I Am Not Thus Perceived—Then Simply Look Above (Up and Back) For The Source Of light, and Hold To (or Yield Into) The Highest Center (or Most Ascended Source) Of the field, Rather Than To what may be perceived to the left or the right.

If The Cosmic Mandala Is Perceived, or If Any Spot or Circle or Shape Of light Is Perceived, Look To Its Center and Be Drawn Upwards (Up and Back). . . .

Let My Avatarically Self-Transmitted Divine Spirit-Current Carry You Upwards (Up and Back) Via The Central Source Of the field, and Do Not Seek (or Hold To) what is perceived on the left or the right. Simply Be Released Into What Is Infinitely Above. If My Avatarically-Born Bodily (Human) Divine Form (or Any Subtle conditional Form That Is Identified As Me or Felt To Be Me) Appears, or If The Cosmic Mandala (or Any Center Of Colored light) Appears, or If My Divine Star (or Any Brilliant, Rather Than Soft or Moonlike, Central White Light) Appears—Let That Vision Carry You Upwards (Via The Center, Up and Back) To The Source-Space Above The Total Crown Of the head.

Preparations in Anticipation of the Death of a Formal Practitioner of Adidam

Following are some practical things which can and should be pre-arranged if it is clear a member of Adidam is soon to be entering the death process. Also see Part One of this guide, "Preparing for the Death Transition".

1. Be sure the Durable Power of Attorney for Health Care is completed. It is important to determine who is legally authorized to sign the Cremation Certificate. In California the Durable Power of Attorney for Health Care (DPAHC) includes instructions about cremation. If you are using a DPAHC which is legal in a state or country where this is not the case, please consider adding the following wording (in consultation with a local legal professional): "My agent is to handle the disposition of my remains. I also give my health care agent the right to transfer, transport, and make any arrangements for my body after death which my health care agent deems necessary or consistent in his sole judgment with my wishes as expressed in this document."

2. Help the dying person handle any unfinished business.

3. Have information on reaching non-devotee family members of the dying person. Encourage the dying person to talk with family about their wishes on how they want to be served after death, if they have not yet done so.

4. Be sure someone has access to all the information necessary for the death certificate (date of birth, state of birth, full name of father and mother, mother's maiden name, and dying person's Social Security number.) The person who has all of this information is called the "informant" and the informant's name will go on the Death Certificate.

5. Know who is responsible for paying for funeral expenses. Get information on funeral home services and discuss costs and procedures with the person who is responsible for these. (Mate Moce does not pay for funeral expenses.)

6. Be sure a doctor sees the person at least every 20 days (or more often if medically required), or whatever the required time is in your state or province that can prevent a coroner's investigation. Be sure the doctor knows Adidam policies and wishes in regard to serving someone who dies.

7. Decide where the vigil will be held and what will need to be done to turn the room into a sacred environment similar to a Communion Hall.

8. Locate a source of dry ice. Know when the place is open and assign someone the responsibility to obtain dry ice within 24 hours after death occurs. Get it in 1/2 inch thick slices, about 10 pounds total—or more if it is crushed.

9. If the dying person is capable of communicating or could do so with assistance, encourage him or her to compose even a brief note to Beloved Adi Da and arrange to have a gift sent.

10. Serve the dying person by doing laying on of hands and the Devotional Prayer of Changes (not for the body to heal necessarily, but for the release of the individual into the Divine or for easing of pain).

Preparations in Anticipation of the Death of Someone Who Is Not a Formal Practitioner of Adidam

Devotees often wish to bring the Wisdom-Teaching of Avatar Adi Da Samraj into service of a family member or close friend who is dying. There is much we can offer, but there is a profound difference when the dying person is in direct relationship with Beloved Adi Da and when he or she is not.

When considering how to bring Avatar Adi Da's Wisdom on death and the death process to a friend or relative who is not a practitioner, consider that individual very carefully. What is his or her Spiritual orientation, if any? Is he or she familiar with Avatar Adi Da? If so, what has his or her response been?

Begin by finding out what has moved and attracted your friends or relatives beyond themselves, even just a little, into the feeling of the Mystery of life. Is it the beauties of nature? If they are Christian (practicing or not), do they feel a strong association with Jesus? With another religious figure? To the Bible? Does music or literature open their heart to the feeling of the Mystery? You may be able to read or tell them stories from the Great Tradition. There may be an opening for sacred music or chant. They may be receptive to simple relaxation exercises to practice "letting go". There are many tapes available to the public now to assist the relaxation and "letting go" process.

You will need to find out and utilize what you can to help draw your friend or loved one out of problematic fear, self-isolation, and doubt as they approach death.

Look for ways to bring Beloved Adi Da's Great Wisdom and Compassion to the circumstance of your intimate's dying process and death. It is always appropriate to bring the Blessings of Beloved Adi Da in the form of His Wisdom-Teaching. Simply remain sensitive and open-hearted to the individual you are serving. (This service may or may not involve explicit communications of a primarily verbal nature, and may or may not directly use Beloved Adi Da's Name or Murti Image. If not, then you will have to be more inventive in your approach.)

Remember that you are not responsible for the way your loved one chooses to die—you should not try to take on their karmic "baggage". Each of us has a unique confrontation to go through in life and in death, and most people will die just as they have lived, although their tendencies may be even more exaggerated. If an individual has not lived a particularly conscious or responsible life, oriented to ego-transcending love and ego-surrender, then it is unlikely that he or she will suddenly do so at death. Be aware of and practice with your own expectations and desires relative to this.

At the same time, however, people can make a remarkable turnabout when faced with their own death. Dying individuals are often far more receptive to such instruction than you would have expected based on their responses when healthy.

Once it is medically established that the person you are serving is terminally ill, be observant of your own and the dying one's egoic tendency to be drawn into the search for cure. Becoming distracted and fascinated by the many options, both conventional and alternative, interferes with the process of self-yielding and release.

On a practical note, find out what your family and friends' wishes are as to how they are to be cared for. Do they want to be cared for at home or in a hospital? What are their feelings about life support, resuscitation, and organ transplants? Have they signed a Living Will or Durable Power of Attorney for Health Care? If not, are they willing to do so? These forms are available from any hospital or hospice. What is their attitude toward embalming and cremation?

Use good judgment about when it is appropriate to talk about death itself. It takes time to adjust to news of a terminal illness. It is often easier for a person to discuss the practicalities of their death (such as legal preparation and funeral directions) than to discuss the death process itself.

Try to interest your friend or family member in the idea that death is a process that occurs over time. Introduce them to the concept that there is a separation of the gross (physical) body and the subtle (etheric) body, and that occurs over a three-day period following the death of the body. Tell them that it is very helpful to be rightly served and guided over this period, so that the process of release can be uninterrupted. At this point, you could discuss the wisdom of letting the body remain as undisturbed as possible, thus avoiding the morgue, autopsy, organ donation, and such. Discuss the three-day vigil and how that could be accomplished.

It may be helpful to anticipate possible conflicts of interest and purpose among family members, yourself, and the dying individual. Yield where you can. The Blessing of Adi Da Samraj that you have known in your own practice needs to be brought into this situation in a harmonious manner. Don't cause conflict or confusion for your loved one and/or family members by righteous or unfeeling behavior. If you find yourself falling into this pattern, take some time out to feel through your own fear and grief and anger to present Happiness. This is the only disposition that is truly serving.

An important preparation for death, which anyone can relate to, is to forgive and be forgiven, as Beloved Adi Da has Told us. If this form of unfinished business is not handled, it will cause the individual to cling to his or her body-mind even as it is clearly dying. Helping the dying person resolve his or her relationships with others can be a significant form of service.

There are two books which can be very useful in helping non-devotees (adults and children) understand Avatar Adi Da's Teachings about death. Those are *What, Where, When, How, Why, and Who To Remember To Be Happy* and Molly Jones's book *The Sky Goes on Forever,* which are available through the Adidam Emporium (1-877-770-0772).

Serving My Brother-in-Law's Passing

A Leela by Eileen Mulvihill
about Serving Someone Who Is Not a Formal Practitioner of Adidam

The following is a Leela, written in the form of a letter to Beloved Adi Da, from Eileen Mulvihill, a longtime devotee of Avatar Adi Da, about serving the death of her brother-in-law, who was not a practitioner of Adidam.

January 14, 1995

Beloved Bhagavan Adi Da, World-Teacher and Heart-Master for all Beings,

All Praise to You and Your Wisdom-Teaching!

For the past five or six years my sister has been going through the ordeal of watching George,* her brilliant scientist husband (of 35 or more years), go through the debilitating decline of Alzheimer's disease, finally ending up in a nursing home on life-support systems. About two weeks ago, she decided (after about six months of disagreement with her children who didn't want the life-support systems removed) to remove the life-support and call in Hospice.

Last week my niece called me in tears and told me her father was dying, voicing her fears, and asked me to go help her mother. It was a three-hour drive to where they live, which gave me time to engage the Devotional Prayer of Changes. My prayer was to remain transparent in my service and allow You to do Your Transforming work for my sister and her family.

Entering George's room, I could feel the fear and hysteria in everyone—my sister, my nephew, my two nieces, and in George. I went over to him, placed my hands on his heart and his head and started talking to him. He was breathing heavily and had a severe case of the hiccups and his eyes were full of fear.

I told him who I was and then said, "George, you're going through the dying process, don't be afraid. There is no death, only change and transformation." (I said that very forcefully at least three times.) "Your wife is here with you, your children are here, and we will be here with you during this process. We all love you and are completely willing to release you to a greater process, release you to freedom from this body and mind."

I started massaging his chest, he started breathing easier, the hiccups went away, and the room became very calm. I could feel Your Presence there; tears of gratitude rolled down my cheeks. I asked my sister to come and place her hands on his head and heart. I whispered to her and told her she should tell him everything she felt in her heart. Then, I asked the "children" to step out in the hall.

* Name has been changed.

After giving them warm hugs and allowing them to cry out their grief, I told them, "We need to make the room very quiet and conscious. We need to remove the mobiles and anything distracting, leaving just the plants, flowers, and music." I talked to them about the process of release and how we needed to allow George's attention to turn to the Divine and not to bring him back with any demands or needs on our part.

The girls quietly began cleaning up the room. My nephew, however, still needed to talk about the life-support issue. He still didn't agree with his mother's decision. Also, having become a Catholic about five years previous to this time, and having married a Catholic woman, he was wondering about bringing in a priest. Based on Your Wisdom, I was able to talk to him about how important it is not to impose one's own religious beliefs on an other, especially during the dying process. I told him it was important to read a dying person readings that coincided with that individual's own faith. I asked him to find readings in the Bible that George would enjoy and to read them to him. Later my nephew's wife arrived. She had a lot of fear about the removal of the feeding tubes. Her fear had taken on the form of anger directed at my sister, and there had been a confrontation between them. Based on Your Wisdom-Teaching and what I had just experienced in serving the transition of my beloved daughter-in-law, Cathy (see pp. 60-67), I was able to calm her down and invite her to participate in serving George's process. She became very cooperative and loving.

During the four-day period, I was able to bring Your Wisdom-Teaching to all family members in one way or another, and the event was being Transformed. We read to George, played the classical music he loved, his wife talked to him from time to time, I did three or four meditations a day at his bedside. Sunday night it seemed that his time was drawing near, so my sister and I and the two girls stayed all night quietly in the room. My attention was on You, my Beloved, and I felt Your Help most profoundly. About 5 a.m. his breathing changed and became short and heavy. Others became alarmed. My sister cried, "He's suffering." "No," I said, "Look at his face. See how beautiful he has become. He is not suffering." It was true. All the swelling was gone from his body, and he looked about 18 years old. His skin was luminous, and his eyes were open and clear. It looked to me like he had already gone, and it was just the body breathing out the last breaths. The hospice nurse was called.

I found a pulse on George's neck, and as I held my fingers there he started breathing slower and slower. His wife told him, "We love you, release you, and we will all be okay. You are free to go." He stopped breathing and the pulse was gone.

Then we straightened out his crooked body, closed his eyes and mouth and made preparations to wash his body. I'd talked to my sister and the girls about how we had served Cathy during her vigil, and they wanted to do something similar. I had brought some holy water. The hospice nurse arrived about that time and my nephew shortly after. We told them what we wanted to do. The hospice nurse made the necessary calls to the mortuary and made arrangements with the doctor and the nursing home, so that we had three and a half hours to wash his body and sit quietly with him saying our good-byes. Each one of us said what we felt about him and told him how much we loved him and read a poem, a passage, an essay, sang a song, or said a prayer. It was very beautiful and extremely Blessed. I felt You there most profoundly, my Beloved, and my tears were ones of gratitude and joy—I think theirs were too.

My sister decided not to have him embalmed. Then, because of the rains, they couldn't bury him for three days, so he was packed in ice and laid undisturbed.

When I left them, the entire family was ecstatic! The girls saw a complete and perfect rainbow on their way to the airport. "See, Dad wants us happy!" my niece exclaimed.

Beloved Heart-Master Adi Da, all during this event I felt You as the Divine World-Teacher! You are here for everyone—anyone who will turn their attention away from themselves to You—in this case, You in the Form of Love.

The hospice nurse asked many questions about Your Wisdom-Teaching. I'm sending her *Easy Death*. She thanked me for coming to help my sister and said, "Before you came it was like a war zone, and then it became very calm and beautiful". I told her, "That's because I brought my Spiritual Master with me."

Beloved Master, may I take You with me everywhere and always. I am so grateful to You and feel so Blessed to be Your devotee. I love You so very much, Beloved. You are the Great, Compassionate, and Loving One. You were my resort this whole past year as I served my beloved daughter-in-law, Cathy, and was so Instructed by You—and now, as if my cup wasn't full enough, You have Blessed my sister and her family in their time of need.

Thank You! I love You, I love You, I love You,

Eileen

Practical Actions to Take When a Devotee Has Died

The following are practical instructions for handling the business associated with the death of a practitioner of Adidam. Throughout all of this practical action, the primary principle is to help the devotee who has died to release all egoic attachments into the Unconditional Reality of Avatar Adi Da's Divine Being. Help them surrender and be open to Beloved Adi Da's Divine Grace and Blessing.

Immediate Actions After Death Has Occurred

1. Report the death of a devotee.

Have your Mate Moce representative, Cultural Services Manager, or Radiant Life Clinic representative notify Beloved Adi Da immediately. Avatar Adi Da will want to know such details as:

—who was with the person as he or she died,
—where the death occurred,
—whether or not the dying person said anything as he or she died,
—how conscious he or she was approaching death, and
—how the deceased is being served now.

Reports should be directed to Charles Seage, who will pass them on to Beloved Adi Da.

2. Arrange for the vigil.

If needed, the vigil coordinator may contact Judy Wendling, Adidam's Mate Moce Director, for guidance.

—home phone (707) 462-8467
—work phone (707) 275-0556

Or call Leone Lewis, a long-time devotee and professional funeral director. She is well-versed in the laws of California, Oregon, and Washington states.

—home phone (425) 712-9836
—work phone (800) 276-0000

A message can also be sent out via e-mail to alert other devotees.

3. Locate the deceased's Durable Power of Attorney for Health Care.

Copies of this document may be with your local Mate Moce representative, your local Radiant Life Clinic, your Cultural Services Manager, or at the home of the deceased.

4. Make arrangements for the cremation.

Have one person—specifically someone who is named on the deceased's Durable Power of Attorney for Health Care—begin making arrangements with the funeral director or crematorium to ensure that all necessary paperwork and scheduling will be handled in time for the cremation.

Other Important Actions:

Keep the body undisturbed.

Try to keep the body completely undisturbed for the first couple of hours.

—If the death occurred in a hospital, ask the hospital staff that you be left alone with the body for a couple of hours. It is preferable to arrange this in advance.

—Try to prevent an autopsy and removal of the body to a morgue. In the case of a sudden death, it will be more difficult to prevent these.

Notifying local authorities.

—If a doctor has seen the person within the past few weeks (three weeks in California), the doctor may be able to determine the cause of death and sign the death certificate.

OR

—If the person has been under Hospice care, you can call Hospice and they will call the doctor and the coroner. No autopsy will need to be performed.

OR

—If the person is <u>not</u> under Hospice care and has <u>not</u> been seen by a doctor recently, a coroner or medical examiner will need to be called. Do not move the body before the coroner arrives.

Prevent invasive procedures.

Invasive procedures are disturbing to the release process. We recommend no organ donation, autopsy, or embalming.

Embalming versus refrigeration.

It is often useful to let the funeral home director know that our request for no embalming is one of our religious principles. Generally, funeral directors won't challenge religious principles.

If preserving the body is a question, firmly request that the body be refrigerated rather than embalmed, even if a funeral director tries to suggest otherwise.

Laws on embalming vary greatly from state to state and from country to country. The best source of information regarding preservation of the body can be found through local licensing and regulatory boards. In the United States, this is called the State Funeral or Cemetery Board.

NOTE: The Federal Trade Commissioner of the United States says embalming is not required unless the body needs to be transported by commercial transportation, or if the funeral home needs to keep the body for viewing for a certain length of time.

Use of a funeral home.

You will need to use the services of a funeral director, generally, to complete necessary paperwork and do the cremation. You may choose to hold a vigil in a private home or in a funeral home. Transportation of the body may be handled by devotees in a van or by a funeral director.

Consider that non-devotee family members may feel more comfortable in a funeral home setting.

If death was due to a communicable disease (Hepatitis B, meningitis, HIV, etc), embalming may be required. It is the law in some states in the U.S., although there appears to be no public health purpose served by embalming. [Referenced from *Caring for Your Own Dead* by Lisa Carlson (Hinesburg, Vermont: Upper Access Publishers, 1987), p. 64.]

Death of a child.

The Durable Power of Attorney for Health Care (DPAHC) is only valid for people 18 years and older. Even if parents state their beliefs and preferences, these have no legal standing when the death of a child occurs. A good relationship with the local authorities may help, as well as the Devotional Prayer of Changes.

The three-day vigil.

The practice for devotees of Adi Da is to perform a three-day vigil after the cessation of the heart-beat. The three-day vigil is a process of purification. Those serving the vigil are there to help the devotee who has died be released to the fullest extent possible. See Part Three for a full description of the process of the vigil.

Cremation.

Beloved Adi Da recommends cremation over burial. It helps if the deceased has already spoken to family members about his or her wishes on how to be served after death. It is very important that the proper written consent be given for cremation (see pp. 14-15).

Schedule the cremation for immediately after the completion of the three-day vigil.

Practical Actions to Take When a Devotee Has Died Unexpectedly

Unanticipated deaths present far more of a challenge than deaths that are expected. Getting control of the situation takes quick thought and action. Circumstances can vary tremendously.

If death occurs in a hospital:

1. Try to keep the body completely undisturbed for the first couple of hours after death. Ask the hospital staff to leave you alone with the body. This can usually be arranged without any problem.

2. Call your local Mate Moce representative or Cultural Services Manager. (See p. 35, points 1 and 2.)

3. In the case of a sudden death, you may not be able to prevent an autopsy. If that is the case, it will at least be useful if you can have the autopsy delayed for as long as possible.

4. Transporting the body. The body may be transported by a funeral director or by a devotee with a van, directly from the hospital to the place where the vigil will be held.

If death occurs outside a hospital:

An unexpected death outside of a hospital is generally the most difficult to handle, and our service will almost certainly be compromised to some extent.

If you are with a devotee who has just died suddenly,

—try to revive him or her if at all possible. You may need to call in a rescue team and have the person rushed to a hospital.

—Hopefully the devotee will have his or her yellow alert card, which gives basic instruction on his or her wishes.

—The devotee's DPAHC may be introduced to hospital staff to prevent extraordinary treatment if there is no clear chance of recovery.

If the person is then pronounced dead in the hospital, see instructions for handling death in a hospital.

When to call a coroner.

If a doctor has seen the person within the past three weeks (exact days vary in different states and countries), the doctor may be able to determine the cause of death and the coroner will not need to be involved.

If foul play or an accident does not seem to be the cause of death, but a doctor cannot determine the cause, a coroner will need to be called. If a coroner does become involved, he or she will probably order an autopsy, which we do not recommend.

Don't move the body before the coroner arrives. The coroner is coming as if to investigate the scene of a crime.

Once the death has been reported and cause of death determined, the body may be transported by a funeral director or a devotee to a place where a vigil will be held.

(For more details, see "Practical Actions to Take When a Devotee Has Died".)

Practical Actions Relative to the Unanticipated Death of Someone Who Is Not a Devotee

Try to prevent autopsy and embalming. As much as possible, try to keep the body undisturbed for the first couple of hours after death, when the greatest activity of energy is taking place.

If you are present with the deceased and there are family and friends who object to leaving the body undisturbed, you might tell them you want to say your goodbyes and prayers privately. They will usually be understanding.

If you are with the person who has died, you can tell the deceased he or she has died and to relax and let go. Even saying these things with the tongue of the mind is effective.

Your greatest service in this case will most likely be to those left behind. Helping them to release their sorrow will also serve the person who has died.

Serving a Death Transition at a Distance

Practitioners of Adidam often call Mate Moce for advice on how to serve a parent or other loved one who has died at a distance. Sometimes practitioners cannot get to the vigil until after the first twenty-four hours, or perhaps they cannot attend at all, and they wonder how to serve the transition of someone who is many miles away.

First, you yourself must understand that the death transition is a process of release, purification, and blessing. Help those who are physically on site with the body to accept this and, if they are open to it, discuss the desirability of avoiding intrusive procedures (such as autopsy and embalming). Tell them it is better to grieve apart from the physical body, and explain why. Help them direct their attention toward releasing the one who has died, and to give that one instructions such as Avatar Adi Da Suggests.

Meanwhile, take the time to feel into your relationship with the one who has died. Mate Moce has found that it may help to look at photographs of the person, or to reread letters to recollect the feeling of that person—you may even want to take these items into the Communion Hall with you. Once you feel connected with the person, turn that relationship over to Avatar Adi Da Samraj and ask for His Help and Grace. Feelingly Contemplate Beloved Adi Da even as strong feelings of your relationship to the newly dead person come up—then practice with these feelings, just as if you were physically present at the vigil. Give that person Avatar Adi Da's Instructions (in brief) in your intention and feeling, and pray that the newly dead person be Helped and Blessed and Released by Avatar Adi Da's Grace. Do the Devotional Prayer of Changes formally to release whatever obstructions may arise, and affirm a graceful transition.

Return to the Communion Hall as often as it feels appropriate to practice the Devotional Prayer of Changes, and perform the Ruchira Avatara Murti Puja for the sake of re-establishing the Beloved of your heart and calling upon Him in your service to the one who has died. Beloved Adi Da has Said that it is good to express our grief and inspire one another with right understanding and right devotion to Him. Allow yourself to grieve and to release and purify this grieving as well. Keep in touch with those at the vigil or attending to the body in order to give them the right orientation and as much of Beloved Adi Da's Wisdom-Teaching as they can accept.

If a fellow practitioner dies at a distance, you can participate in the same way through your own feeling-Contemplation of Avatar Adi Da Samraj and your Devotional Prayer of Changes to bless and release that one.

PART THREE

The Death Transition

Part Three of this guide focuses on descriptions of the changes in the body during and after death, how to care for the body, and how to conduct the three-day vigil. It also discusses ghosts, grieving, and memorial services.

What Death May Look Like and How to Serve These Changes

This section is a discussion of some progressive secondary or observable signs of the withdrawal of energy from the physical body, including practical responses when these signs appear. Note that these signs may not all be evident and some may be far more obvious than others. These signs may also come and go and are not listed in any sequential order.

1. Mottling of the skin or loss of color and sensation from the hands and feet of the dying person.

You can check for this by feeling these areas. At this time, they will be cool to the touch and lose their normal flesh color. The nailbeds of the hands and feet will become darker in color. (In dark-skinned individuals, this phenomenon will be more difficult to observe, but you should be able to feel the changes in skin temperature as well as observe the discoloration of the nailbeds.) Strength and sensation will leave the affected areas and, at some point, these areas may actually seem to be dead or lifeless. When this occurs, the individual will usually be in the final hours of life.

2. Upward turning of the eyes.

A characteristic upward rolling of the eyes will also be noticed at this time, particularly when the dying person is sleeping or drifting out of outward-directed consciousness. You may also notice that the dying person may sleep with one or both eyelids partially open. The luster of the eyes will diminish during this period.

3. Communications of "out-of-the-body" experience.

Some people begin to have, and communicate about, out-of-the-body experiences as they are dying. The relationship between the subtle body and the physical body is greatly weakened at this stage, so it is very natural for these experiences to occur. Certain individuals may see and communicate with the forms of people who have passed away. At times, the dying individual may drift in and out of such experiences and may feel that he or she has already died. In this case, the individual may not be able to distinguish this world from his or her experiences of other worlds. These experiences, though not generally understood properly, do occur quite often in dying individuals.

4. The gradual subsiding of outer awareness.

As a dying person's energy and attention begin to ascend, he or she will appear less interested in and also, perhaps, less capable of engaging in outward-directed communications. One moment such a person may be talking with you, the next moment he or she may seem to slip into a trace-like state in which his or her attention is very withdrawn, and the individual may appear to be oblivious to his or her surroundings and circumstance. Eventually he or she may slip into a coma and die in an apparently unconscious state, or he or she may die fully conscious and capable of engaging in outward-directed activities to the last moment. This second possibility is less common, however.

Regardless of the degree of a person's apparent awareness of his or her surroundings at the time of his or her death, it is always best to presume that one can fully communicate with a dying person. This is true even if he or she is in an irreversible coma due to severe brain damage. It is very difficult to assess an individual's psychic state. Even if a person seems to be lost in a profound coma, he or she may on the subtle level be fully conscious and capable of being communicated with.

5. Fevers and sweats.

There is a common belief that the body heats up just before death. To some extent, this belief is true. Many dying individuals do experience febrile (feverish) and diaphoretic (sweaty) bodily states. These are usually due to the presence of an infectious process or to irritation of the brain's temperature control mechanism in the dying process.

However, the death process is usually one of "cooling down". One of the most obvious signs of life in the body is heat—living bodies are warm. But, as the subtle body of the dying person withdraws, the source of this heat is also withdrawn. When the complete separation of the subtle body and physical body occurs, the physical body begins to cool down and it dies.

6. Weakening of and/or difficulty in breathing.

The breath cycle reflects the presence and degree of energy and life in the body. It is also the principal means whereby the body conducts the elemental exchange necessary to keep it alive. It is only natural that you will see changes in the breathing patterns of those nearing death. These changes will vary from individual to individual and depend mostly upon the person's ability to consciously engage and submit to the death process.

For example, a dying person who is having difficulty with this transition will often use the breath as a way of clinging to his or her body and life in this world. This effort causes a breathing pattern that is forced and labored. You may be able to help by placing your hands on the person's chest and instructing him or her to breathe with you. At first, you will want to copy the person's breathing pattern and then slowly bring it down to a calm and easy pattern. Tell the dying person to relax and follow your example.

Regardless of how well a person is able to cooperate with the death process, as the individual comes closer to death he or she will usually cycle through what is known as "Cheyne-Stokes" breathing. This pattern may be based on the changes in the body's chemistry that occur as the death process advances. The Cheyne-Stokes breathing pattern is characterized by periods of apnea (absence of breath movement), followed by increasingly rapid breathing cycles that climax and then taper off until another period of apnea occurs. At first, this may only occur when an individual is asleep. However, this pattern will eventually characterize all his or her breathing as he or she approaches the critical stage of the death process.

Not all individuals display the Cheyne-Stokes breathing pattern. If it does not appear, you will see a gradual and rhythmic fading of the breath. Just before the breath ceases, it often becomes a gentle gasping with long pauses, until it fades altogether. For others, the breath may become very noisy and labored, as secretions (which are no longer being eliminated) begin to pool in the lungs. There are many variations, but these are the most common.

7. Signs of major organ failure as physical death approaches.

As the body continues to shut down, there will be signs of major organ failure. There may be cessation of urine flow, irregularities of heart rhythm, accumulation of fluid in the tissues, sluggishness (or looseness) of the bowels, and congestion of the lungs.

Moving Out of the Physical Body

As previously indicated, this phase of the death process is active but short. It begins when the heartbeat and respiration cease and ends when the brain begins to die (some four to six minutes later). During this period, the transition out of the physical body to the subtler dimensions of existence begins.

You will observe the following signs at this stage of the death process:

■ **The heartbeat and breathing will cease.** This is the dramatic moment usually presumed to be the "moment of death". In truth, it is simply a milestone along the way. As you will understand from your study of the death process, true death occurs after separation between the physical body and the etheric body completes itself. Until then, life-energy still inheres in the body. The dying person is still capable of being resuscitated and brought back into association with the physical body.

■ **The body's musculature will relax entirely.** When the heartbeat and respiration cease, the dying person's energy and attention rapidly ascend. This is accompanied by the spontaneous relaxation of the body's musculature. The body of the dying person will immediately fall into a slump if the person is not in a lying down position. Occasionally, a dying person's body stiffens immediately when the heartbeat and breathing stop, but as the life-force leaves the body, it gradually loosens and relaxes. Sometimes, at the time of physical death, the bladder and/or bowel will eliminate if they are filled to any extent. It is also possible for a person to have a few random and spontaneous breaths over the seconds and minutes that follow the cessation of the heartbeat and then to grow still and relaxed.

■ **There will be a significant loss of color and heat from the physical body.** During the first few minutes after the heartbeat and respiration stop, you will notice a rapid change in color from flesh-tone to pale straw or a grey pallor (even with dark-skinned people), as well as a loss of body heat. These two life signs, color and heat, won't fully subside until the end of the next stage of the death process, or the moment of true death.

■ **After the cessation of vital signs (or what is conventionally referred to as death), you may notice a sense of "presence" or feel other energy phenomena.** The dying person's release from the physical body, along with the spontaneous ascent of energy that naturally occurs at death (especially in the case of someone who cooperates with the death process), releases tremendous energy into the environment. This release of energy can be felt by those who are present with the dying person as a definite sense of "presence", or a feeling of great peace and calm surrounding and pervading the immediate environment.

If you stand by and observe the flesh body die, you will no doubt experience your own reactive emotions. You may feel shocked that it looks so strange—that "one moment the person was here, and now the person is gone". You may feel an array of emotions and also the uncanny sense that you are not alone. People commonly do the wrong things at this most critical time. One of them is to act as if "it's all over" when in many ways the critical transitional phase of the death process has just begun and your service to the individual who has just died must intensify in earnest. This is not to say that you need to shut out your feelings, but it is very important to discipline your action.

■ **The newly dead person is experiencing a rush of very stimulating higher brain-core phenomena such as loud noises, colors, lights, and fast movement. All of this can be very disturbing and confusing. This is the time to give your instructions clearly and strongly to the deceased.** It is optimal to keep the room and the body undisturbed for the next few hours when your instructions are most crucial. Speak directly into the ear and remind the individual to look up and to the center of any vision that may be appearing before him or her. Remind him or her to release upwards and not to be distracted by visions, lights, and sounds. Chant Beloved Adi Da's Names or forms of the Ruchira Avatara Naama Mantra and have those who are present in the room be steady in their feeling-Contemplation of Avatar Adi Da or engaged in simple prayer (for those who are not formal practitioners of Adidam). Tell the newly deceased what is happening—that death is occurring and that he or she is exiting the physical body. Tell the individual that there will be a transition during which he or she must keep attention very centered and focused. This will ease confusion. Encourage the dying person in his or her release process and upward focus.

Avatar Adi Da has addressed our tendency to employ the popular death movement's tools for "going into the light" or trying to guide another individual to do so. There is a psycho-physical movement associated with the death process, and we need not guide anyone into "the light". On pages 26-27, see instruction #11 and the subsequent quotation from *The Dawn Horse Testament*. Basically, we guide the person who has died to surrender to Avatar Adi Da Samraj and not to be distracted from that devotional surrender.

Avatar Adi Da has also Explained that there is no inherent victory in "entering into the light" because we don't have the ability to hold on to any experience after death, and, unless attention has been transcended at its Source, through sadhana, we automatically start falling into lesser conditional states. What occurs ultimately after death is created by the karmic tendencies which remain.

In April 1991, Avatar Adi Da Gave the following Notes:

AVATAR ADI DA SAMRAJ: To achieve a superior or ultimate destiny after death, an individual must have the ability to transcend mind and the limiting tendency of attention. So, after death, an individual's destiny will be determined by the tendency of his or her mind and attention. That is the way it is. Divine Liberation is a matter of most perfect transcending of the mechanism of attention and the mind altogether. Therefore, it requires most perfect transcending of desire, or the motives of attention. There can be glimpses of sublime things and attractive light in the death process, but, first of all, that in itself is not Divine Enlightenment in the most perfect sense, and secondly, the ordinary individual has no capability to keep attention in that sublime condition after death. And so there is a drifting into the lesser conditional states via the lesser conditional tendencies of the mind.

■ **There may be psychic communications from the newly deceased.** Psychic communications in the form of thoughts, dreams, or visions may occur more often with individuals who have not been prepared to cooperate with the death process or who have died suddenly. This type of communication may be genuine, in which case it is usually an indicator that the individual needs further help in releasing the contents of his or her life.

Sometimes, however, the dead person's intimates (who most often experience these phenomena) are only experiencing their own process of release, which may, in fact, not be directly related to the deceased. It is necessary to bring discrimination to these experiences. Avatar Adi Da has recommended that we do not become distracted or focus attention on these phenomena, but remain in a surrendered disposition, focused in our feeling-Contemplation of Him.

Care of a Devotee's Body after Death

Refer also to the section on serving someone who has died (pp. 35-37). This particular section will cover practical details on preserving the body for a three-day vigil.

Handling changes in the body after death.

After death, the body often will involuntarily empty its bladder or bowels. The blood is no longer circulating, so it settles to the lowest point in the body. Some parts of the body may swell a little. Fluids may be discharged from any orifice. Try to keep the body undisturbed for at least 1/2 hour and preferably 2 hours, as Avatar Adi Da has Indicated the greatest activity is occurring during this time. It should, however, be moved to the vigil site soon after that (no longer than 3 hours after death) as rigor mortis sets in. It is acceptable shortly after death to gently arrange the body in a more relaxed posture, closing the eyes and mouth if you choose, but handle it at all times in a respectful manner. If you tie up the jaw with gauze immediately after death or place a small towel roll beneath the chin, the face will set more naturally with the mouth closed.

Choosing a vigil site.

Holding a vigil in a devotee's home allows much more freedom for the devotional practices of Adidam. If the person died in his or her own home, holding the vigil in the bedroom might be best, so there could be minimal disturbance to the body. Read further on how to prepare the room (p. 51).

A regional Communion Hall is another possibility if there are other places for people to meditate during the three days of the vigil. The room that is used is greatly empowered during this process.

A funeral home may be used as a vigil site, although service will generally be compromised. Devotees will probably feel less free to do puja, chant, and express their devotion to Avatar Adi Da in a public space. And it may be difficult, or at least quite expensive, to continue the vigil through the nights in a funeral home.

Beloved Adi Da has Told us that Sanctuaries are not to be used for vigils unless a devotee actually died on a Sanctuary. Also keep in mind that nearly always some non-devotees attend a vigil.

Moving the body.

Before moving the body, it may be placed on a plastic liner or in a plastic body bag (which you may obtain from the funeral home) to catch any draining fluids and put in a cardboard or plywood casket. It may be left in this casket during the vigil and cremated in it as well, or you may choose to lay the body on a cot or bed for the vigil. When moving the body, if you are using a cardboard casket, it is best for it to be placed on a piece of plywood or a door, preferably with handles (for easy carrying). When laid down at the vigil site, the head end should be elevated to prevent bodily fluids from accumulating in the head region. Bricks or a 4" x 4" piece of wood can be placed under the head end of the plywood. If the head cannot be raised in this fashion, put two pillows under the head to keep the head and shoulders elevated.

Preparation of the body.

You will need:

- rubber gloves
- a few cotton balls and packing tape
- an adult diaper
- 1/2" slabs of dry ice (each slab wrapped securely in plastic—it can cause serious burns) or blue ice packs

Hopefully a Radiant Life Clinic representative or a Mate Moce representative will be available to help you prepare the body. If you are managing the vigil without the help of a Clinic or Mate Moce representative or a mortician, simply wash and dress the body. It would be best for two people to do this together. The washing can be done quickly with lukewarm water. Yerba sante tea, rose water, and saffron water are other possible washing solutions. Using disposable gloves, a cotton ball may be inserted into the anus and held in place with packing tape and/or an adult diaper may be used to collect any draining fluids. A condom or the finger of a rubber glove may be put on a man's penis to catch any draining fluids. Use a deodorant powder on the whole genital area. Then dress the body in a loose fitting garment or simply cover the body with a nice blanket or cloth.

Apply ash and holy water to the body's ajna center (the point between the eyebrows) and heart region. You might want to place the deceased individual's mala or sacred jewelry on the body. You may wish to place an ash packet next to the heart of a loved one who is not a practitioner if you feel confident that this gesture will be well received. Beloved Adi Da has Asked that devotees be wrapped in a "transition shawl" during the death transition and cremated in it. These shawls are to be made by Sacramental Services at Adidam Samrajashram (Naitauba). The transition shawl is to be worn each year during the Mummery enactment and Da Ashvamedha Fire Puja, as well as at practice transition initiations and the death transition. Then the body is to be wrapped in the shawl before cremation. This orange shawl is larger than retreat shawls and is made of lightweight, natural fabric.

The body must be kept cool, so keep a window open or use air conditioning in warm weather. Dry ice in a plastic bag should be used especially over the abdominal area to retard decomposition. (Cold moves in a downward direction so put it on top rather than under the body.) Also use dry ice over any draining wounds. If dry ice is not immediately available, blue ice packs are very helpful. They don't melt, and stay cold for quite a while. Keeping the vital region of the body very cold helps immensely in preventing loss of bodily fluids.

Note about dry ice: Buy about ten pounds in about 1/2" slices. Do not touch it directly, as it will burn skin. Use pot holders to handle it, and wrap it in plastic when you put it on the body. Store it wrapped up in a freezer. It will evaporate rather than melt. Someone should check the ice on the body at least once a day and add more when necessary.

Preparing the room.

Remove all medical equipment and supplies and any other unnecessary items. Keep the room cool. A Murti of Avatar Adi Da should be in the room, preferably one large enough so the Ruchira Avatara Murti Puja can be performed. Have puja supplies available. Leave space in front of the Murti. It is preferable to have the body to the side of the Murti rather than right in front of it as people's attention should be on Beloved Bhagavan Adi Da. Keep enough light on to be able to read. Purify the room with incense and holy water if available. You may also place sage in baskets around the room and mist the sage regularly with water—this helps to keep the air fragrant. Have plenty of incense and candles available.

If a cardboard casket is being used in the vigil, you may choose to wrap a sheet around it or cut a sheet in half and drape the box with it so it looks nicer.

Readings.

Have a copy of *Easy Death* and this Mate Moce Guide in the vigil room. Provide an orientation for those serving the vigil outside the room, so they will be prepared to properly serve when they enter. It is also nice to have some flowers available outside the room for people to offer as gifts when they enter. Gifts should be offered to Beloved Adi Da's Murti, not the body, although some flowers may be placed around the body if desired.

The Three-Day Vigil

The following is a summary of Avatar Adi Da's Instructions for the vigil.

The three-day vigil is a process of purification.

Those serving this event are there to help the dead person move through the lower levels of attachment and to be released to the fullest extent possible.

Keep the circumstance around the body visually and psychically clear, undisturbed, and calm, so that the process of release and purification can take place most effectively.

For this reason, only a few people should serve the vigil at any one time, though occasionally there can be a larger number.

In the vigil, one should sit quietly in feeling-Contemplation of Beloved Adi Da. He Says, "Sit in Contemplation of Me, not the dead person." Release the dead person and whatever arises.

It is fine to make note of any signs that appear psychically, but do not abandon the formality of the vigil. Persist in the process of release. Even if everyone senses the person who died is "gone" or fully released, the vigil should still be carried out for the full 72 hours. (A vigil for a baby could be accomplished in a shorter time, as babies are less attached to their bodies. See pg. 88. The same applies to animals.)

Formal recitations should be done from time to time throughout the vigil from Avatar Adi Da's Wisdom-Teaching.

The recitations should be appropriate for the occasion. Readings from traditional literature should not be done during the vigil. Readings may help the individuals conducting the vigil to relate to the death process as Beloved Adi Da Recommends and, therefore, serve their process of release.

In the early portion of the vigil, it is useful to occasionally tell the deceased "Relax, let go. It's all right." If the death was sudden, it is especially important to tell the person that he or she has died, as such a person's confusion about what is occurring may last a lot longer than someone whose death was expected.

One may also read Beloved Adi Da's formal Instructions on the death process into the dead person's ear (see p. 26). Give instructions slowly, firmly, and clearly. Keep in mind the deceased is experiencing all sorts of confusing sights and sounds, so we need to keep our instructions simple and clear.

In the case of devotees of Avatar Adi Da who have died, a Murti of Adi Da should be placed in the room where the vigil is to be held and it should be appropriately served.

There should be a ceremony every day associated with the Ruchira Avatara Murti Puja and a ceremony on the last day just before taking the body to be cremated.

There should be no picture or memorabilia of the dead person in the room.

Also, those attending the vigil should not address the dead person by his or her name. This would tend to draw the dead person to maintain association with his or her body. The one who has died is no longer the persona he or she once were and should not be reminded of that persona.

Soft chanting may be done periodically throughout the vigil.

The formality of the vigil is maintained for the purpose of rightly focusing everyone's attention in the process of release.

The dead person is addressed compassionately yet in a formal manner. If this is not done, those individuals who are both serving and attending the vigil will tend to lapse into their own cycle of grief and/or fascination.

As a service, those serving the vigil should relieve grieving family members and intimates of practical responsibilities relating to the vigil, including physical care of the body.

Those who are heavily grieving should be helped to regain their balance. ("Conscious exercise" and instructions relative to breathing, to balance strong emotions, and use of recitations relative to transcending grief would be helpful. For further instructions on breathing, see Appendix D, "The Discipline of the Breath", in *The Scale of the Very Small.*)

Beloved Adi Da has said that grief is a natural and useful activity that releases the one who grieves as well as the individual who has died. Expressive grieving is part of the release process, though it should neither interrupt nor interfere with the vigil itself. For this reason, family members and those intimate with the deceased who are in the midst of this grieving process are served to regain their balance by members of Mate Moce and other devotees, apart from the vigil itself.

Involving non-devotee relatives and friends of the deceased in a vigil.

Expect to have non-devotees attending the vigil. (In fact, someone needs to be sure family members have been informed of the death if the one who died had no partner or family nearby.) It is important that each devotee talk with his or her family members about his or her DPAHC and funeral arrangements, so everyone will know how we wish to be served after death.

Since devotees often live in cooperative households rather than nuclear family settings, it would be helpful for household members to set aside a place for everyone to keep names and phone numbers of their next of kin so these people may be contacted in case of serious illness or death.

Family and other non-devotee friends should be oriented to the purpose of the vigil. You might tell them that Avatar Adi Da Says that it takes approximately three days for the etheric body (or spirit if they would understand this) to completely separate from the body and that we are serving that process of release in performing the vigil. Whatever you may say, non-devotees are nearly always moved by the peace and caring that is evident during a vigil. If non-devotee intimates wish to spend time alone with the body, allow them to do so, but once they leave the vigil room, the devotee attending the vigil should intensify the instructions to the one who has died. The deceased will probably have been drawn back into association with his or her body by the presence of such an intimate, so it may be useful to tell him or her that their intimate will be all right and it is okay to release and let go. Wave incense, chant a form of the Ruchira Avatara Naama Mantra—realign the person who has died to return his or her attention to Beloved Adi Da.

It is important to avoid conflict with families. Compromise is more important than righteously upholding our way of doing things if it may cause conflict.

Keep in mind that conflict and hurt feelings during a vigil are likely to draw the deceased back into association with his or her body. As stated earlier, the vigil should always be carried out in a disposition of calm. This is more important than procedural matters.

The final Puja.

A final Ruchira Avatara Murti Puja should be done at the end of the three-day vigil. This is an excellent time for a celebration of release for a larger group of devotees. Mate Moce recommends inviting particularly good chanters and priests and everyone who has served the vigil. In addition to the puja and chanting, this occasion could include recitations from *Easy Death* or other parts of Avatar Adi Da's Wisdom-Teaching, special sacred music offerings, and Leelas of Beloved Adi Da's Work in the life of the departed devotee. Make it a true "celebration of passing".

Cremation.

Ideally, immediately after the last puja, the body should be transported to the crematorium. This could even be part of the closing celebration, with chanting continuing as the body departs. Try to arrange for the cremation to be immediately thereafter, as sometimes bodies are not cremated for days after being delivered to a crematorium. Transportation may be handled by a funeral director or a devotee with a van.

Ashes will be available a day or two later. Request that all the cremains be returned. Sometimes the body will not be fired sufficiently to burn the large pelvic bone to ash. Practitioners should ask that any bones not turned to ash be pulverized and added to the cremains.

Scattering of ashes.

As part of serving the dead person's release, the body is burned to ash, so there is no body to be attached to. To further serve this release, the ashes should be scattered rather than kept in an urn somewhere, as the being may even be drawn to that location.

Avatar Adi Da Samraj has Instructed that ashes should not be scattered on the Retreat and Pilgrimage Sanctuaries or their peripheries. Sanctuaries are places that need to be purified of spirits and attention on the dead. Ashes should be scattered in a natural area or in the sea. Check local laws about where scattering is or is not allowed.

A Note about Ghosts

In the following Talk, Avatar Adi Da explains how to help beings who have become ghosts in the death transition.

AVATAR ADI DA SAMRAJ: Just as the recently dead can be helped by their friends reminding them of what is going on when the physical body is dead, so also those recently dead who are locked into the etheric and who are what might be called "ghosts" can be helped. Those individuals may not be present in the physical plane all the time. They may pass into unconsciousness and then return again. They may go into some field of subjective reverie, and it is in that plane that they experience what could be called "hells" and difficulties and strange frustrations, like strange dreams. Then they may again return to association with the physical plane while they are yet in the etheric body, invisible to most others but perhaps even experienced there.

Some of you may have had experiences with such individuals, perhaps people you knew and whom you experienced in this way shortly after their death. I have had contact with many such individuals. They can be released by associating with them very much as you would associate with someone who is alive right now. You must help them be aware of their actual situation, because they think they are still physically alive. They have not quite figured out their situation. It is a problem to them. They are not in a normal state. They are emotionally shocked and agitated, strangely attached to people and places.

The one major thing that is going on with them is that they are not aware they have died. They think they are alive, and yet something about their situation does not quite make sense to them. They cannot get people to respond to them, and the people who are in the rooms that used to belong to them act as if they are not there. Yet they move around, and they do things like everybody else. They could sit and watch TV with you at night. They could hang out in your rooms, watch you have sex, even try to have sex with you.

The one thing you can do to help them is to make them aware that they are dead, explain what has actually happened to them, and describe the next step of their relinquishing, relaxing, letting go, moving on. Such direct address to these individuals, if you have some perception of them, can be useful to them. (July 3, 1987) [*Easy Death*, pp. 280-281]

Grieving

In the following excerpt, Avatar Adi Da Addresses the process of grieving for an individual who has died.

AVATAR ADI DA SAMRAJ: Ordinary people live to fulfill the physical dimension of existence. Therefore, they are shocked and disturbed by death. They want to forget death. They want nothing to do with it. They are only totally threatened by the death of another, and they typically experience extraordinary grief.

In itself, the grief of being separated from the company of another is natural. But debilitating grief, grief that prevents you from associating with the one who has died, that prevents you from releasing that person and serving his or her continued process of relinquishment—such grief is not good.

You must be prepared for your own death, and you must be prepared for the death of others. You must serve others once they have died, because they have not disappeared nor ceased to exist. You do not want them to become ghosts, trapped in the etheric body, so that they roam in this world for decades and more before they are able to pass on. You must serve their ability to notice their condition, relinquish it, and move on from the physical.

Mourning (perhaps that is not even the best word for it—the celebration of passing is perhaps a better way to describe it) should be a process whereby the person who has died, or given up the physical, is given the opportunity to notice that fact and to see that all his or her friends and relations also notice it and know that he or she has passed.

In the Way of Adidam, all those participating during the vigil should remind the individual, through prayers, affirmations, and reading My Wisdom-Teaching, that he or she is undergoing a process of letting go. They should point out the next step and encourage the person to relinquish the physical and move on. (July 3, 1987) [*Easy Death*, p. 281]

Memorial Services

Death ceremonies of all kinds are practiced throughout the world and are important in meeting the emotional needs of the survivors. A funeral is a service held in the presence of the body, with either an open or closed casket. A memorial service is held after the body has been removed and tends to be more positive than a funeral because it focuses on the life and values of the person who has died rather than on the dead body.

It is important to be aware of the difference between a memorial service and a vigil. During a vigil, the focus is on helping the person who has died to release all attachment to body and mind and everything in his or her life. So bringing out old pictures and sharing memories would only serve to draw the being back into association with the body. But others have a need to celebrate the person's life and share their grief, and this can be done at a memorial service. As stated above, memorial services should not be held until after completion of the three-day vigil and the cremation.

There is not a formal written memorial service in the Way of Adidam, but occasions have spontaneously occurred after some devotees' deaths and have been very useful.

Holding a memorial service a day or two after the cremation is an excellent time for people to come together. A memorial service was held after a devotee died in Lake County, California, in 1998. Pictures and articles from his life were displayed. There was a formal meeting in which everyone was invited to recount their favorite memories about their friend. Some told Leelas about this devotee's relationship to Beloved Adi Da, while others told about the delicious food he often made. Non-devotee family members and neighbors were present and were very moved by all the love expressed.

A memorial service could include music and readings. It might include some inspirational writing by the person who has died, if this is available. People attending can be asked to share their thoughts, feelings, and memories.

PART FOUR

Leelas

These inspiring Stories of Avatar Adi Da's Service to dying individuals and their intimates serve as wonderful illustrations to the points described in this guide.

The Illness and Transition of Cathy Lewis

Told by Her Intimates and Friends

Cathy Lewis came to Avatar Adi Da in 1974 when she was in her early twenties. For two decades, she served as a missionary and cultural leader in Adidam. She was well-known for her devotional relationship with Avatar Adi Da, and she inspired many others in their surrender to Him. Cathy, her intimate partner, Jack, and their daughter, Sukey (who was twelve at the time of Cathy's death), lived in the northern California region near the Mountain Of Attention. Throughout her life, Cathy suffered from narcolepsy (a condition characterized by sudden brief attacks of deep sleep), but had otherwise never shown signs of serious illness.

In December 1993, Cathy had a series of seizures and was admitted to the hospital. She was diagnosed with a virus infection in the brain, and it was thought that it would clear up within weeks. However, further testing indicated there was a tumor and that surgery would be necessary. In February 1994, Cathy underwent brain surgery and the tumor was found to be worse than expected. The doctors gave her six months to live (without treatment) and perhaps three to five years with chemotherapy and radiation.

Jack describes the early period of Cathy's illness.

JACK: The vision of my intimate having such a struggle physically just broke my heart, over and over again. For me there was always the impulse to try to do something about it while at the same time I knew there was nothing I could do, that I had no means, ultimately, to be able to do anything—but still I tried to do whatever I could.

Avatar Adi Da was notified of Cathy's situation early on, and we received Instruction from Him about what to do and what not to do. Avatar Adi Da's Instruction to Cathy was essentially that she should prepare for her death and release everything to the Divine, including any expectations about how long she might live. He Said that the acceptance of the inevitability of death is fundamental to the practice of the Way of Adidam, and that she should surrender her concern and live a real life of retreat for the remainder of her life. Beloved Adi Da also Asked the devotee physicians advising Cathy to make sure that they kept in mind the quality of her life altogether, and not simply get into a desperate search for bodily survival at any cost.

I saw in Cathy a growing resort to Him that was really heart-breaking. Cathy took Beloved Adi Da's Words to heart, but she was also still very hopeful, especially at the beginning of the year, that something was going to work—that there was going to be a miracle and everything was going to turn out all right. But it became clear that something else was occurring, and she more and more came to terms with the process of the body dying. It wasn't just that the body was dying, but that its functions were falling away: the capability to remember, to speak, to walk and maintain balance. She had to watch and experience her functional being disintegrate. But while all this was going on, she was becoming increasingly surrendered at the heart and loving to everyone who came to see her. She continually gave love and energy to people—it blew my mind.

Many alternatives to conventional treatment were investigated, and Cathy spent time in Texas at a clinic that employed an experimental method of treatment with a more impressive success rate than chemotherapy and none of the side effects.

In July, Cathy developed an infection and was again hospitalized. She rapidly dropped into a coma. Her condition was critical, and the doctors were not certain that she would pull through. After several days, she opened her eyes and began talking again. She related an experience she had had during the time that she had been so critically ill.

CATHY: I went into another world. This other world was an ecstatic world where people were full of God; that is the only way I can describe them. There were at least twenty people there, two of whom I recognized as devotee friends of mine. I was in a state of total physical inability, and I would move from that into a place that was totally Happy. It was very blissful and easeful to go into this state where these people were. There was this feeling of Happiness running through this place, and I just felt totally Happy to be aligned to them. I would close my eyes and fall into this place. Then I would wake up to some degree and say to myself, "I am supposed to wake up! I am supposed to wake up!" But I could not really wake up. I didn't have a way to wake up, so I would close my eyes and go back into this place of Happiness. I don't know how long this went on, but it seemed like a long time. The only thing going on was this Happiness.

When I did start to be awake and alive again, everything had changed. I had let go of my concern. I just let it go! All these people in this place of Happiness had helped me.

When Cathy was released from the hospital, she tried other alternative healing regimes, but in October, the results of a brain scan revealed that the tumor was growing.

Jack's mother, Eileen Mulvihill, describes an incident with Cathy on October 24:

EILEEN: One day, Cathy said to me, "I am getting worse, right?"

In my fear, I became angry. "That is the wrong message to give your body!" I said. "Why don't you just say 'To hell with this cancer. I am not going to do cancer anymore!'" I hit the table with my fist. Cathy began to cry, and I began to wail. Emotions we both had been holding back all year seemed to burst forth. Soon we were both wailing and hugging each other.

"Let's go to the Communion Hall," I suggested.

We sat in front of Adi Da's Murti, and I confessed all my fear, anger, and sorrow to my Beloved Master. It was obvious that I was clinging to Cathy, not willing to surrender this human relationship that had given us all so much delight. It was also obvious that I had to let go of that clinging and release her to her process.

When I stopped talking and wailing, Cathy looked at the Murti and began to speak very clearly to Adi Da. She said over and over again, "I just want to be with You, I just want to be with You."

In that moment, we both knew we had to give up our search for a cure.

The next day, October 25, Jack and Cathy received Notes from Avatar Adi Da:

AVATAR ADI DA SAMRAJ: The conventional orientation of people with a terminal illness is the search for a cure, as if cure will happen. I specifically Instruct My devotees not to indulge in this point of view. Of course, there is reason to look for treatments that are therapeutic, and such treatments are fine, but the conventional point of view is typically the "I am going to be cured" mentality, rather than the release of all negativity and surrendering in heart-Communion with Me.

My Instruction to Cathy was to handle her life-business, make arrangements for her daughter, relinquish her household arrangement with Jack, and enter into a life of retreat and intensive religious practice and renunciation. She has done this to some degree, but she has also been coloring her life with the search for the magical cure and social religiosity. She should obviously correct this. Her disease has reached the point where cure is unlikely, and it seems that she cannot be expected to live much longer. Therefore, she should handle her life-business, make arrangements for her family, and enter into a renunciate life in preparation for her transition.

She should release all negative thoughts. She should not try to go on with business as usual. It is fine to have the support and all the help of her friends and family and My devotees. Very possibly there may be remission of the disease and some continued life. Yet, in any case, her life should be a life of renunciation and meditation, the handling of life-business and relinquishing of life-bondage, so that she is prepared for this transition.

She should know that there is no death. The body dies, but the subtle components continue and these must be purified and transformed. Therefore, she must do the purification of the subtle and do the transcending work in the time that remains in her body. This means she should rightly maintain celibacy and live in a circumstance where she can maintain her days in meditation, puja, study, chanting, practice "consideration", and discussion wherein life-business is handled and life-bonding is relinquished.

Through this right practice she must relinquish the exterior part, the anxiety and the fear of this transition, so that she is fully prepared for it when the time comes. She must let go of the exterior part without any disturbance or reluctance. She should neither be meditating on dying nor affirming dying. She should release all negative thoughts. If she continues to have some lifetime, fine, and if she dies, fine—that should be her point of view. In other words, her time should be spent in her practice as My devotee, and her practice must become profound instead of life-oriented and socially oriented. The more profoundly she purifies and transcends her own limits with her remaining time in the body, the more profound her transition will be whenever it finally comes.

Does she know the seriousness of her present condition? The facts of her illness should be presented to her before this Instruction of Mine is given to her, so that she is ready to receive it. This should be done with others around her—Jack, the doctors, the cultural servers, and Mate Moce. All these people should be aware of the service she requires now, and they should know what they must also change.

The same people must decide how to communicate to Sukey on the basis of her maturity. They should deal realistically with her, so that she can also be prepared. I assume adults are assuming full responsibility for her. She should have such support. Cathy will not be able to release her until she can see that Sukey is in a right and positive and happy situation and that she will be able to deal with Cathy's transition.

Cathy should not get into any morbid or negative disposition relative to all of this. She should be real, straightforward, profound, and not negative or morbid. Death is a real process, a process that must be really and seriously embraced. She must prepare for it and maximize auspicious signs, and so must the people who are related to her.

How anyone rightly prepares for death is an individual matter. In some cases, it may be better for the individual to remain more active, and in others not so. Yet even those who remain more active should assume the renunciate form of life and disposition, and increased meditation. It is fundamental to the religious process that everyone release life-bonds, and such release is fundamental to the process that precedes the transformation that is death.

There are three important things My devotees must do altogether in the Way of Adidam, and these same three things are to be maximized before the death transition: (1) handling life-business, (2) practicing renunciation, and (3) living in a way that maximizes heart-Communion with Me. This basic Instruction from Me should be given to all whose life may be brought to an end before too long. [October 25, 1994]

Eileen describes the reception of these Communications:

EILEEN: Adi Da's Words were completely wonderful and Liberating. They were full of Compassion and Instruction for all of us, and we felt His Blessing Power and Transmission. Cathy cried, I cried, Jack cried. We knew the search for cure was over, and we had to do something entirely different. We knew we had to resort to Beloved Adi Da.

A dramatic change was able to occur. We were no longer trying to beat death, but were cooperating with it. It was after these Notes that Cathy was able to let go of Sukey and Jack and allow the community to make plans for taking care of them. After that point, she was truly resorting to Beloved moment to moment, and as a result was Given the most incredible Blessing and Help from Him.

Beloved Adi Da's Notes were also read to Sukey. She received them very well, finally understanding what she had been feeling all year. Her life would change—indeed had already changed—and would never be the same. She cried, and expressed her anger at the situation, but was able to express clearly what she felt she needed and wanted in her life. I was impressed with her courage and maturity. This was liberating for her, and she seemed brighter afterwards.

Sukey moved next door with one of her friends. Members of Mate Moce and Cathy's friends and family tended to Cathy's now extremely simple life. She kept a Murti of Adi Da by her bed, and even when her friends would turn her so that she might be more comfortable, she would often turn back so that she could regard Bhagavan Adi Da's Murti Form. Many of Cathy's friends came to see her from all over the western United States. She seemed bright, and would always find a way to let those who visited her know that she was saying goodbye to them.

JACK: In the last week or two, I stepped back from my practical care of Cathy, and the community of devotees stepped in, which was really wonderful. The gift of community in the Way of Adidam is wonderful. I was so grateful for everyone's help throughout that whole time. Everybody just stepped in and started serving Cathy, helping her in every way you can think of, and making it possible for her to let go and also enabling her to be in a heart-sphere. She lived the last week or so in this circle of love. Friends of hers from around the world called and some came in person to say their good-byes.

Avatar Adi Da was informed regularly of Cathy's condition. When it was obvious that the end of her life was near, He sent special Gifts of Blessing to Cathy.

EILEEN: On November 10, we received word that Avatar Adi Da was sending His own shawl and some sacred Gifts especially for Cathy, and that these would be brought back right away by Fiona Syme, a devotee returning from retreat at Adidam Samrajashram. Fiona arrived on the 12th in San Francisco, where a friend met her and drove her up to Cathy's house. The gifts were presented to Cathy formally: She was wrapped in our Sat-Guru's beautiful orange shawl, and her body was anointed with ash and holy water He had Blessed. Flowers He had Blessed were placed on Cathy's head and heart. The occasion was filled with our Beloved Guru's Heart-Transmission.

JACK: In the last days there tended to be a mood of solemnity and concern, and that was hard for me. But late one evening, two of her lady friends and I were sitting in the room with Cathy and started telling stories about how crazy she is—because she is. She is a wild, crazy person. So we just started remembering times with her and telling these stories. It was like a party.

So we just got into this party mood with her, telling stories until about midnight, and then everything came to rest. Her friend Mary stayed in the room with her, and I went out into the living room and lay down. I was half asleep when Mary came out and said, "I think Cathy is about ready to die. Her breathing has become very, very slow. I think she's dying." Just as she said that, the phone rang. Someone was calling from Adidam Samrajashram to say that Beloved Adi Da was asking about her at that moment. Immediately an intense wind began to blow. I felt that the wind was a sign.

Cathy died within minutes after that phone call and the beginning of the wind.

While Cathy's body was washed and arranged for the vigil, devotees at the Mountain Of Attention Sanctuary were awakened to gather and engage the Devotional Prayer of Changes for Cathy's auspicious transition. Word was sent immediately to Adidam Samrajashram and relayed to Beloved Adi Da.

The three-day vigil for Cathy began. She was wrapped in the orange shawl that Beloved Adi Da had Given to her. Her room was decorated with flowers. Devotees from northern California took two-hour shifts to read Adi Da's Wisdom-Teaching aloud, chant, and meditate with the body.

JACK: The vigil was a wonderful process—very, very graceful. I think everybody who participated in the vigil felt very quickly that Cathy was tremendously relieved. That's what I felt.

Even though everything that had occurred was graceful, it had also been a profound struggle. During the last period of her life, when the body and its functions were deteriorating, it was just a struggle. The body wasn't a good place for Cathy to be anymore, so there was a relief from all that.

At the end of the three days was the final puja blessing Cathy in her transition. Many of Cathy's friends attended, and the occasion was full of Adi Da's Blessing.

When the vigil began, Adi Da sent a message to devotees that they should be sensitive to any communications from Cathy during her time of transition—especially any feeling that Cathy was having difficulty leaving the body-mind. Just after the final puja was finished, Jack received a message from Dennis Dardzinski, a longtime devotee living in Marin County (a two-hour drive from Cathy's home). Cathy had appeared to him in vision just after her passing, and had also seemed to want Dennis to convey a message to Jack. Later, Dennis recounted his entire experience.

DENNIS: I was studying Beloved Adi Da's Teaching at 7:45 Thursday morning, the 17th of November. This was after my morning meditation, and I was sitting on the couch in the living room. As I sat, I felt a sense of relief go through my body and Cathy appeared to my internal vision and she seemed relieved and happy. I did not know for sure, but I felt that Cathy had probably died. On Tuesday, we had heard that she had been given twenty-four to forty-eight hours to live. I had talked to Jack at that time, giving him my love and energy.

At about 8:00 a.m., a local devotee called and said that Cathy had died at 2:00 that morning. I went into the meditation hall to offer a prayer for Cathy. Immediately, I felt Adi Da's Presence strongly and was drawn into an internal scene in which Cathy appeared. She was moving through a great process of energy. She seemed tentative about the process and its tremendous force. She was frightened or confused, but she seemed to be trying to figure out what was next. She made contact with me for help. I reminded her to relax, release, and find our Sat-Guru. I repeated this single instruction for a while. At one point I noted Cathy animating her characteristic quality of "Wow, look at this! Really?!" relative to the process. At some point, she thanked me for my help and implied that she would also have to release this help connection. I reminded her to let go and release—Sukey was okay. Jack was okay. And she had been a good devotee.

Next I observed Avatar Adi Da as this Unlimited Force, Radiant but Discernible as Him, and Cathy as this small force, a white-ish being moving toward Him. There was an Embrace, a Union. It impressed me as Adi Da Being Shiva and Cathy Shakti, or Krishna and a gopi. This was the impression I got. It was ecstatic! I called out loud: "Yes, that's it!" Cathy was loving her Heart-Master. Cathy was a Bhakti of God. Then Cathy appeared as a white-ish being. She was full, happy, intelligent, and confident with her love relationship to Avatar Adi Da. She was on the other side now, beyond anything of her former life. It seemed she wanted me to communicate this to Jack. Let Jack know she was okay, beyond anything that Jack may feel about the "wrinkles" in their relationship—any guilt, crankiness, being ripped off, and so on. She seemed happy and full.

Only five minutes or so after Jack received the message from Dennis, the phone rang. Adi Da was asking again if anyone had received any kind of communication from Cathy!

◆ ◆ ◆

JACK: It had been a very graceful process with Cathy altogether. I didn't feel like I had anything left to work out with her, any emotional difficulty. There had just been a tremendous expression of love. But when she was gone, all of sudden I felt this pain at the heart. It surprised me. I didn't think I would feel it. I felt a pain, an intense loss, and I also felt kind of dead, as if something in me had died. People would tell me it was the grieving process. I didn't actually expect it because everything had been simple and graceful.

Then at some point Beloved Adi Da invited Sukey to come to Adidam Samrajashram, Adi Da's Hermitage-Retreat in Fiji. That was completely wonderful. I was so ecstatic that she would be able to come and connect with Him, because that was the main thing I wanted for her.

That night I had one of the most profound dreams I've ever had. In the dream, I was being invited to go to an initiation performed by devotees in Hermitage. The initiation was being held at a very primitive place, a little stone house. It was archetypal. I remember looking around and having eye contact with devotees, and there was just the sense of Beloved Adi Da, pure Communion with Him. That was the only thing that was happening. It wasn't a remote place—there were even cars going by. But inside it was just like going back to a primeval space. One woman that I have known for a long time was bringing out fabric that had been in Beloved's personal environments. First she showed me a beautiful piece of white fabric and then brought out a beautiful crimson fabric, then beautiful orange fabric. It was incredibly potent.

Right in the midst of this dream, there was a knock at the door which woke me up, and I was told to call Hermitage. I immediately knew that it was an invitation. When I called, a devotee who had just come from Beloved Adi Da's Company said that Beloved had asked for me to come to Hermitage with Sukey.

At this moment, I was just broken up—heart-broken in gratitude. It was the answer to what my heart was praying for.

The night Sukey and I arrived at Naitauba, I was invited to a gathering with Adi Da. I went into the room and prostrated, and everyone immediately made room and gestured for me to go up front. I went up in front of Avatar Adi Da and bowed down, and started to embrace Him. He's so Beautiful. He's just there, and is so round. I was holding His arms, and His face was so big. There was so much emotion, I didn't know what to say.

I muttered something about Cathy, and He Said, "Sh, sh . . ." It was clear that He knew everything about what had happened. There was no need to tell Him anything. He Said a couple of things in the interchange that confirmed that He knew everything. It was obvious in the feeling.

I just kept feeling how soft He was, the roundness of His face, and I looked into His eyes. He kept Telling me that it was all right. He said, "Cathy is all right." He Said, "She's with Me." And He would point at Himself and Say, "She came to Me." He must have Said that a dozen times while we were talking.

A couple of times, I started to say "Cathy was . . .", referring to her in the past tense. The first couple of times, He Said, "No, she <u>is</u> with Me". Then I think it became clear that I was still not getting the point, so He got a little fierce with me, and Said very clearly, "She is with Me! She is looking at you through these eyes."

I knew that was true. I had known that when she died, that she had gone to Him. It was clear. There was nowhere else that she was going to go. But just to hear Him Say it washes the heart. He just kept Saying it over and over again, "She is with Me. She is here." And He pointed to His Heart on the right.

He Said I looked really old. But it wasn't just that. He Said, "I know that it's been hard. I can see it in your face. I can see how much you've aged this year, and it's all right. You did everything that you could do. You have nothing to feel bad about." He rubbed my face, rubbing the wrinkles out of my face.

He also Spoke to me about Sukey. He Said He was going to take care of her. That meant so much to me, because I've seen how difficult it had been for Sukey. In some ways, it was harder for me to deal with that than with my own grieving. I just really wanted her to connect with Him. He Said that He was going to take care of her. He Said, "I'll see her tomorrow." I told Him I was so grateful to Him for that, and expressed something about how I felt it had been very difficult for her. He said, "When she sees My face it will be all right."

SUKEY: When I found out that Cathy, whom I loved and love very dearly, had brain cancer, I went into shock. I tried to forget about it. Naturally, this was impossible. Because she was so sick, I hated being at home. I tried everything to get out of the house, so I did not have to feel the sorrow. Cathy felt unloved now, and Jack felt abandoned by me. I tried to make myself feel better with food and making "cliques" with different friends. Then Cathy got really sick, and I left the house to live with one of my friends.

On the morning Cathy died, I rushed over. She was lying in bed, very pale, with an orange shawl that Beloved Adi Da had Given her wrapped around her. I cried, not knowing what to do.

Then Beloved Saved me. He invited Jack and me to come to Hermitage on retreat.

One night, we knew Beloved was coming to gather with us at Hymns To Me. When He arrived, Beloved Adi Da walked up onto the porch where we all stood. I was right in front, so I could see Him very well. He took me in His arms and Said, "Your mother is all right." He kept repeating this and looking straight into my eyes. "She is with Me now and she loves you very much. She has told Me so, many times. Did she tell you how much she loves you before she died?"

"Yes," I said.

"Good. She loves Me, too."

All the while He was holding me close to Him, healing my heart. I kept saying, "Thank You."

Then He Said, "I hate death. That is why I am here, so I can bring everyone to Me when they have died. Cathy is with Me. She is so happy. She loves you, like she told you. She is listening to us right now, My baby. Right now. I will always take care of you, and Jack will take care of you. All your life, I will take care of you. I Love you."

"I love You too, Lord."

Then He walked inside, and I followed. I was invited to sit next to Beloved on a big divan. He looked over at me and Said, "She did not leave you alone. She left you with Me. Do you understand?"

"Yes, Beloved."

"You are a very mature girl to understand what I am Saying—very mature. I mean it. Cathy didn't want to leave you. She was forced to. She is very happy now with no narcolepsy and no disease in her head." Music was playing and devotees were dancing, and He Asked me to get up and dance for joy, so that is what I did.

Later in the evening, I sat next to Beloved again on the divan. I moved behind Him and rubbed His back for a long time. He turned around and Said, "Does she love Me?"

"Yes, Beloved," I said, "I love You." And He Gave me a kiss.

Beloved Healed my heart from all of the shocks. He Broke my heart truly. He Told me to love Him, and Remember Him always and to love Him. I love Him so much. I bow at His feet in joyous praise and love.

JACK: That first night on retreat, I felt that my grief and sorrow about the loss of Cathy was healed on a basic level through Beloved Adi Da's Grace. One of the things He Said was that Cathy's process was easeful. He Said, "I made it easeful. It could have been terrible." And it was truly easeful. It could have been very, very difficult. But she experienced very little pain or discomfort, and the process was quick. Her mother has been a hospice worker for years, and she said it was the most easeful death she ever saw.

Avatar Adi Da Said, "I did that for Cathy." And He looked at me and Said, "I'm going to do it for you when you die. I'm going to do it for all My devotees."

The Greatest Gift of My Life: The Leela of Hien Lam's Passing

by Carmen Morrow

On June 13, 1997, Hien Lam, a devotee of Avatar Adi Da, passed away as a result of breast cancer. Hien, a Vietnamese of Chinese descent, was born in Hanoi in 1944. She lived through the Vietnam War, describing it to her daughter, Minh (or "Carmen", as she is known to her American and Canadian friends), as the most terrifying experience of her life. Hien risked her life to bring her parents and most of her nine siblings out of Vietnam, and after the war was over she worked as a refugee counselor for the United Nations. It was 1988 when Hien first discovered Avatar Adi Da Samraj. Eight years later she had become His formal devotee, and her heart's desire was fulfilled in November of 1996 when she was able to speak to Avatar Adi Da in an occasion in which He responded to questions from devotees. Shortly after this, she discovered that the breast cancer that had first appeared in 1995 had returned, and she was eventually hospitalized. This is the story of Avatar Adi Da's Service to Hien, told by her children in 1997. Carmen Morrow, then 22, and a recent graduate of film school tells most of the story, and Joshua Gildart, then 9, whose father and Hien's husband, Ron, is also a devotee of Adi Da, concludes with a confession.

CARMEN: A few weeks before her death, my mother told me that her first true sight of God was in the vulnerability of a Vietnamese refugee she met who had lost all his family in the war and was completely stripped of all his possessions and all his intimates. Her response deeply impressed me and explained her many years of studying traditional Asian religious and Spiritual paths. Coming from a family of devout Buddhists (particularly my grandmother), she was always sympathetic to Buddhism, but when she came across Beloved Adi Da's Teaching she was immediately attracted to Him. She read His Teaching for many years, and then was moved to become a devotee; she was a devotee for the last year of her life.

The biggest joy in her life was when she talked to Beloved Adi Da on His Birthday in 1996, telling Him she would be His devotee forever. It broke my heart. My mother had been through many difficulties in her life, and when Beloved Adi Da Gave her nothing but Blessing and Appreciation during their conversation, it released me of all my concern about her. I knew that Beloved Adi Da would take care of her, even in her illness and her death—which He has.

When the cancer reappeared, it had spread to her liver. She was in a great deal of pain and underwent six months of chemotherapy, which reduced but didn't eliminate the cancer. In the last week before she died it spread to both her lungs.

I had been trying everything to find a cure for my mother. I spent all my time, from the minute I got up to the minute I went to bed, doing something to try and help, whether it was researching alternative cancer therapies, talking to health professionals, or just being with her and doing "the laying on of hands" [a simple healing practice] as it is taught in Adidam, or reading to her from Beloved Adi Da's Teaching. I was really desperate, and one night, as I was going to visit her at the hospital, I began to feel how desperate I really was. I had been suppressing it by keeping busy, trying not to feel how painful it would be to lose her.

I resorted to Beloved Adi Da in that moment and asked Him, "What do You want me to do?" And I actually heard His voice: "Bring her to Me." It was very strong and very adamant. Naturally, I took His words literally. I knew that Beloved Adi Da was in Los Angeles. And I knew that if I could get my mother's energy up enough to make a trip, she could see Beloved Adi Da.

I went in to her room. She was sleeping. It was early June now. Before she woke up, I did the laying on of hands for her and I Invoked Beloved Adi Da. I felt His Love. It was a very Fiery and Fierce Love. When I did the laying on of hands for her, Beloved Adi Da's Energy was so strong that my mother's body would shake wherever I laid my hands. It was a very ecstatic evening for me because the whole room felt really strong with Beloved Adi Da. Afterwards, I just held my mother until she opened her eyes. And the first thing I said to her was, "Mom, we're going to see Beloved."

She had the most radiant smile. It was completely open and happy. Even though she was weak, bedridden, on I.V., she just beamed, and said, "Really?" And we talked about it. I went home that night, and the next morning, even though the circumstance was conventionally bad, I was happy. I put on some music in my room, and I danced while regarding Beloved Adi Da's picture. I was so grateful for His Intervention. I went to see my mother every day. I decided that I would go down to Los Angeles first and arrange a circumstance for her and then I would come back and get her.

My brother Joshua, who was nine years old at the time, and has always had a remarkable devotional response to Beloved Adi Da, had always called himself "Mom's pilot to Beloved". Even as a very young child he always said to her, "I'm your pilot to Beloved." So, as I was preparing to go, I went in and said, "Well, Mom, Joshua's your pilot, and I'm going to be your flight attendant." My mom gifted Joshua with a little pilot's hat on his birthday, and whenever he saw Mom he wore that.

Everything had changed since that night I had simply asked Beloved Adi Da for Help. Whenever Joshua and I went to see my mother, we dressed in our best clothes and were very aware that we were there to serve her, and to serve her Contemplation of Beloved Adi Da. I told her that the only thing she needed to do was to feel that she was in a bubble of Beloved Adi Da's Presence. We made formal agreements with all the devotees who came to visit her that they were only to bring Beloved Adi Da to her—to read His Teaching to her, and to feel Him deeply when they were around her. We filled her room with beautiful pictures of Beloved Adi Da and lots of flowers. It became a bright and happy place. I sensed in my meditations that I should only read to her from *Four Thorns Of Heart-Instruction* [the original edition of *Hridaya Rosary*], and *The Dawn Horse Testament*, and we did that. It was actually a wonderful and ecstatic time. I would just go in and find myself in such a deep feeling of Beloved Adi Da, just happy. It was very intimate and very special. Without my even realizing it at the time, He had Gracefully led me to fulfill His Admonition to "bring her to Me."

Within a week, I went down to Los Angeles, the devotees were very helpful. But after two days I got a call and everyone at home was saying that my mother had gotten a lot worse and that her pain was almost unbearable. She was on maximum doses of morphine and other pain killers. It broke my heart to hear that my mother was in so much pain. When I sat in Darshan [an occasion of formal sighting] with Beloved Adi Da for the first time down in Los Angeles, I was the first person He looked at. In the middle of the Darshan, I saw a tear roll down His Face. And I realized that I was trying to be brave and that I was suppressing a lot of pain. And so I just cried, too.

By the end of the Darshan, what had impressed me was that it actually didn't matter if my mother survived this cancer or not. And that was very hard for me to accept. I wanted her to be alive. I loved her utterly. But Beloved Adi Da showed me that it didn't matter because she would be with Him either way. I understood that I was to serve Beloved Adi Da and serve my mother and that that was the same thing. That was a tough thing for me to take. It was very humbling. But I knew that this was real, that it was true. I couldn't just ignore it, I had to accept it. By the end of that Darshan, in my Contemplation of Beloved Adi Da, I had reached a state of equanimity. And my reactions, emotions, desires in relation to my mother—all the content about all the things I felt I needed to do—subsided. In that particular Darshan, Beloved Adi Da's body became gold and "Bright".

The Truth that He Communicated to me was not consoling in the ordinary way. It was "heat", a fiery Transmission of Truth. It was like He was purifying my personal attachments and desires and preferences at great speed. It wasn't soothing at all! His Eyes became like two headlights, looking right into the depth of who I am.

That was on Wednesday, June 11. At 5 o'clock in the morning on Friday, I got a call with the news that my mother had passed away. It was such a shock. I went into my room and regarded a photograph of Beloved Adi Da. I wept, and then I prayed to Him to take her. I knew I had to surrender her—as hard as it was, I knew that was the only thing that I could do in that moment. And, after that, when I thought of my mom and felt her spirit, I felt she was happy. I could hear her voice saying, "I'm with Beloved, don't worry." She had such a wonderful, loving, humorous quality to her voice when she spoke—very pure and happy.

I definitely wanted to see Beloved Adi Da before I went home. At the Ashram, the women there embraced me and put me on retreat. I spent the morning reading *Easy Death* [Avatar Adi Da's book on the process of death and dying], and sat in the meditation hall. Soon a devotee came in and said I had an important phone call. Beloved Adi Da had invited me to come and sit with Him right away, so that I could go home immediately to serve my mother. I was beside myself! I was so happy that I forgot to be sad. The whole day was such a paradox. Someone asked me what I wanted to do before Darshan. And I said that I wanted to go and get a nice frame for the photograph of my mother so that I could present that to Beloved Adi Da. Even on such a weird, tragic day, I felt so happy. I bought a rose, and I went into a card shop and tried to find an appropriate card. None of them struck me until I saw one that had a Chinese character for luck on it. That was the only one that suited the circumstance. And I wrote inside, "Beloved Adi Da, although I'm crying, my heart tells me that You have Given me the greatest Gift of my life. Thank You. May You know that my brother and I are forever grateful to have the good luck of being your devotees. We love You." I pasted my brother's and my photos inside the card, cut out in the shape of hearts. I got dressed, had a bite to eat, and then it was time to go to Darshan.

I was invited to sit in the library, where two devotees spoke with me about myself and my mother. I felt wonderful in that environment with those women, I felt very relaxed. Then Trivedi Naamleela, one of Beloved Adi Da's daughters, came in and gave me a hug. Then Adidama Sukha Sundari came in and told me that Beloved Adi Da had Asked that I offer Him a gift and then massage His Feet, so that I could receive His Transmission in that way and bring it to my mother, to serve my mother's body. I was heart-broken. I had already been Given so much, and now Beloved Adi Da was Giving me another Gift. [In the traditions, the

Guru's Feet are revered as a point of particularly potent contact with the Guru's Blessing, and devotees worship the Guru there.] I was immediately nervous, and I asked Adidama Sukha Sundari to show me how to massage Beloved Adi Da's Feet. And she did, by massaging my feet.

Then, while I waited downstairs, Adidama Sukha Sundari went up to answer Beloved Adi Da's questions about my father and Joshua's father. Finally, it was time to take our seat in the main living room. There were about ten women or so. I was given a place right in front of Beloved Adi Da's chair.

Beloved Adi Da came in, and took His Seat. He looked at me, and the first thing that He did was raise one of His eyebrows. I just beamed. He brought me into relationship with Him, just like that. He was so Attractive, and He had such a beautiful look on His Face. And He was so very close to me. I offered the gift of my mother's photograph, the card, and the rose. I thought I was to offer my gifts at His Feet, as everyone always does, but Beloved Adi Da put His Hands right out and took them all. I was heart-broken again.

He first gave my mother His Regard for quite some time, looking at the photograph. Then He set it aside and took the rose and set it aside. Then He opened the card and read it, quickly, and set it aside. And then He immediately put His Arms out. I couldn't believe it. I walked right into His Arms and just held Him. I was ecstatic. Beloved Adi Da held me very firmly. He really held me close and tight. And then the loss of my mother started to pour out. I sobbed and I heaved, nestled in His shoulder. And I just kept breathing Him in.

I felt how utterly Compassionate Beloved Adi Da is, how "human" He is. In a sense, it felt so ordinary. And yet I could feel Him taking all of the sorrow into Him and making it possible for me to surrender to Him. It wasn't an effort at all, because He Loved me. I could feel how much He Cared about me, personally, and for my whole family. I was so touched by His Attention and the Gift of His Embrace. He held me for a long time. A long time. And even when I felt that He would let me go, He kept holding me. And when my tears subsided, and my breathing came back to normal, I whispered spontaneously, "Thank You, thank You, I love You, I love You." And He Said, "Tcha, Tcha." ["Tcha" is Adi Da's special sound of Blessing.] At last, He began to release me a little bit. And then finally brought me right in front of Him and wiped my tears with His thumb. Then He took my mother's photo and pressed His thumb on her head, between the brows, and on her heart. In that moment, I felt that Beloved Adi Da completely understood the intimacy between my mother and me. It was as though He was demonstrating to me, "This is the wound of love, this is what it feels like." It was the sweetest gesture and a complete surprise. My eyes welled up again, and I sank back into His Arms. After some time, I had exhausted all the tears and thoughts about what was happening, my breathing became normal, and I could only feel Him. It was the most sublime moment of peace and infinite love. At the perfect moment, Beloved Adi Da gently pulled me to face Him. He wiped my tears again and kissed me on the cheek. I prostrated. I was just shaking—my body was literally saturated with gratitude. I was moved beyond any other thought or feeling. I only felt utter gratitude and love for Him.

When I got up, I remembered I was still invited to massage His Feet! His Gifts seemed to be endless! I approached His Feet, and I looked to Adidama Nirvanasati Hriddaya, who gave me a nod. I began with His right Foot, doing the most conscious, loving, sensitive massage that I could. All of my worry and nervousness about doing it right was gone. I was so in love, I <u>am</u> so in love with Beloved Adi Da, that in that moment I felt that I was like one of Krishna's gopis—just absolutely loving Him. And loving every inch of His Foot.

It felt like a release. I could feel that I was also performing this service for my mother, expressing her devotion. I was heart-broken by the sacrifice Beloved Adi Da makes being Incarnate, "in" a body, and Enduring and Absorbing and Purifying everything. After I finished massaging His Feet, I moved back and took my seat, Contemplating Him. When He looked at me again, I began to cry again—out of happiness and gratitude and also grief, all at the same time. His Eyes were watering, too.

Then Beloved Adi Da picked up the photograph of my mom and handed it to me. Again, I was totally surprised, and overwhelmed at the thought of receiving my mother as a gift from Him! It touched me so dearly, as though He were truly Showing me that whatever loss and pain I surrendered relative to her death He had transformed and returned to me in the form of an eternal heart-relationship with her. He was literally demonstrating that the Divine completely transcends death. I immediately prostrated for this mind-blowing Gift.

All of this had taken about twenty minutes. Then Beloved Adi Da picked up the card and got up and went right upstairs, very purposefully, as though He had Work to do.

I prostrated and all the women embraced me again. Soon, water and ash and a pink rose and a cookie that Beloved Adi Da Blessed for my mother came downstairs. I was told that they were for use on my mother's body. Before I left, Adidama Nirvanasati Hriddaya gave me a hug and explained that there would be a photo of me hugging Beloved for me and a photo of me massaging Beloved's Feet for my brother, when they were developed. She also said, "Don't worry, Beloved is taking care of her."

It was a two-hour plane ride to Vancouver and the whole time the memory of Beloved Adi Da's embrace was still very tangible. I could even smell Beloved Adi Da's cologne on my shirt! I was in a state of bliss. Just beside myself, so in love, just so in love, and so happy.

When I came home, there were about twenty people there, including my mother's entire family and all the local devotees. "No wonder Beloved held me for so long!" I thought. It was obvious that I was to bring Him to them as well, and to allow their sorrow to be released to Him through me. Even though they weren't all His devotees, it was just human surrender to the Divine. I hugged everybody with intensity and real attention.

Seeing my mother's body for the first time was extremely difficult. Although I had always understood the body as being a vehicle for life-force, the sight of her made me truly recognize this. She was no more than a "lump of elements", as Beloved Adi Da Says. Nonetheless, she had a beautiful and surrendered expression on her face which seemed to ease any concern in me.

The next morning, I woke up at about four o'clock, full of fear and even panic at the thought of having to see my mother's body again. I turned to Beloved Adi Da and surrendered it, feeling a sensation on the right side of my chest that felt like Beloved Adi Da taking His Seat in me. As soon as the sun rose, I walked to the beach. I was still Contemplating Beloved Adi Da, and I literally felt the Mystery of God. I could feel the Mystery in everyone and everywhere, in every weed, every grain of sand, every wave, every molecule of water, every little bit of me. And that was my mother, and that was Beloved Adi Da, and I felt very happy. It was such a relief. Later that day my brother and I performed a special ceremony on my mother's body. I touched her body with the water that Beloved Adi Da had Given her. And I pressed the ash on her forehead, on her ajna chakra. It was sign of release.

In meditation, I heard my mother's voice say again, "Minh, I'm right here."—as if she were saying to me, "Come on!—it's no big deal." I felt her spirit right in my heart. She said,

"Live, be free, be happy." I had surrendered my mother to Beloved Adi Da, and He had placed her right back in my heart, tangibly. I felt her kisses, I felt her embrace. I felt Beloved Adi Da was my mother, and my mother was Him. In my deepest heart-feeling, there was no separation.

I still miss my mother, and there are times when I really wish she were here—in person. But I know that on the day I lost my closest intimate, I gained my Closest Intimate. I feel so profoundly moved by Beloved Adi Da that I can't help but want to live my whole life in devotion and service to Him. He is the most primary Love.

The next week, on the eve of Beloved Adi Da's departure for Fiji on July 5, Carmen brought her brother to Los Angeles, where he, too, received Beloved Adi Da's Regard, outside the home that had been Beloved Adi Da's residence for several weeks.

JOSHUA: I was amazed. He was so Beautiful and so Blessing. It made me feel very happy. I felt like I'm the luckiest boy in the world. When He came out, He looked at all the other people first. After that, He looked at me and Carmen and smiled. He was standing two or three feet in front of me. Then He came up to me and Touched me on the top of my head with His right Hand for what seemed like a couple of minutes. It felt very Strong and Loving. I felt that He was Giving me Love and Happiness, so I don't have all the suffering and bad moods and unhappiness. Then He leaned over and Kissed me on my temple. I've never felt better in my life. I felt, "Thank You for taking care of my mom."

"Feel Me Infinitely Above and Shoot Straight to Me Like an Arrow"

A Leela of Lance Barham's Blessed Death
in the Deathless Company of the Incarnate Divine Person,
Avatar Adi Da Samraj

by Deborah Fremont-Smith

Lance Barham was a devotee of the Divine Heart-Master, Avatar Adi Da Samraj, for fourteen years. He died in November 1998, at the age of 39. When he died, Lance had been suffering for two-and-a-half years from Lou Gehrig's disease, a terminal illness that attacks the nerve cells and pathways in the brain that lead to the spinal cord, eventually resulting in total paralysis of the body. In the process of dying, Lance was drawn—by the Grace of his Divine Guru—deeply into the real practice of Contemplating Avatar Adi Da Samraj, and was progressively liberated from his fear of death and even his sense of mortality.

Lance had two important qualifications for receiving Avatar Adi Da's Blessing Grace: He loved his Beloved Guru, and he trusted Him. Through that love and trust, he was Blessed with the capability to surrender more and more deeply into a profound acceptance of the Divine Mystery of Existence Itself; and so his death was transformed from a morbid, fearful event to a sublime passage that was full of the Sign of Avatar Adi Da, the Victorious Love-Bliss of Eternal Being.

The story of Lance's relationship with Avatar Adi Da is an inspiring example of ego-transcending Spiritual practice, of outgrowing the limits of the mortal self in heart-Communion with the Divine Person. And it is also a demonstration of the process of Divine Grace that is always available in the Company of Avatar Adi Da Samraj. We all are dying; and, if we can allow ourselves to truly feel our mortality, we will also feel our heart-need for the Divine Person, Who is Greater than death, and Who Calls us to Awaken as Him.

◆ ◆ ◆

Lance was born in the Yukon Territory of Canada, in the town of Whitehorse. His mother was single, and he spent much of his early childhood in the care of his maternal grandparents. (During the early 1960s there wasn't a great deal of social tolerance for unwed mothers in that small community.) Lance's father was part Lakota Sioux. Their relationship was strained, and he would never know his father well, but they did have some contact over the years. It was through this connection that he gained familiarity with Native American customs and rituals. Lance's affinity and reverence for the natural environment seemed grounded in his Native American heritage.

Lance was a big man, full of vitality. Self-educated, a landscaper by trade, he was famous among family and friends for his irreverent humor. He lived in Europe and Israel for six years, and when he returned to Canada from overseas he settled in Nelson, British Columbia.

It was there, in the mid-eighties, that he met his intimate partner, Robin Melville, and her four children. There was a group of Avatar Adi Da's devotees in Nelson who met weekly at her house. Robin describes Lance's initial encounter with his Divine Guru:

ROBIN: Lance came one night with a mutual acquaintance. He was about to become a student of a Tibetan Spiritual Master, but he took one look at Beloved Adi Da's Murti and he knew. That night he told me, "This is my Guru."

In June 1996, about two months after his 37th birthday, Lance was diagnosed with Lou Gehrig's disease, and was told he had between 2 and 5 years to live. Robin remembers how shaken the doctor was at seeing such a young man, so likable and full of vitality, receive a death sentence.

ROBIN: Lance and I, the doctor, our family and friends—we were all devastated by this news, which came entirely without warning and was a total shock. Lance and I came home from the doctor's appointment and just lay down on the bed, and cried together in a long, serious embrace. This was the real deal coming down!

In April of 1997, almost a year after he was first diagnosed, Lance and Robin made a trip to the Mountain Of Attention Pilgrimage and Retreat Sanctuary in northern California for the Celebration of the 25th Anniversary of Ruchira Avatar Adi Da's Teaching-Work, and to see their Divine Guru. Lance would take his last unaided steps on the Sanctuary. In June, he would need a walker and by mid-summer a wheelchair.

Shortly after returning to Canada, Lance told Robin that he had had a profound experience of receiving Avatar Adi Da's Blessing in the form of His Descending Current of Love-Bliss—the movement of His "Bright" Spiritual Transmission of Divine Consciousness and Energy into the body-mind of the devotee through the top of the head.

In one of the many letters of thanks Lance wrote to Avatar Adi Da Samraj during the course of his illness, he describes the feeling of receiving Avatar Da's Current of Love-Bliss:

Thank You for Your Precious Gift of Darshan. Your Beauty Attracted me beyond all my physical dilemmas, and I was able to surrender and feel Your "Brightness" Descending through me, Pervading me, Surrounding me. I felt You so strongly that my head pressed back and I felt You Flooding my being with "Brightness". I felt utterly Pervaded by Your Graceful Blessing Light. You are the Giver of All Bliss and Happiness. I am so grateful to You, My Beloved Guru, for Your absolute Blessing Gifts.

This experience changed Lance's orientation to what was happening with him. The search for healing came to an end, and Lance began to concentrate himself in the relationship with Avatar Adi Da.

ROBIN: He began writing beautiful poetry about Beloved Adi Da, and talking about Him more and more. In the past, he had read Beloved Adi Da's Word to us, but now he did so more often. He was giving himself over.

There was one Essay by Avatar Adi Da that Lance particularly loved; he would recite it and speak of it often throughout his illness, and referred to it on his death bed. The Essay, titled "The Heart of Understanding", is the prologue to *The Knee Of Listening*, Avatar Adi Da's Spiritual Autobiography. It begins:

Death is utterly acceptable to consciousness and life. There has been endless time of numberless deaths, but neither consciousness nor life has ceased to arise. The felt quality and cycle to death has not modified the fragility of flowers, even the flowers within the human body. Therefore, one's understanding of consciousness and life must be turned to That Utter, Inclusive Truth, That Clarity and Wisdom, That Power and Untouchable Gracefulness, That One and Only Reality, this evidence suggests. One must cease to live in a superficial and divided way, seeking and demanding consciousness and life in the present apparent form, avoiding and resisting what appears to be the end of consciousness and life in death.

Before his formal sightings of Avatar Adi Da in April of 1997, Lance had been very involved in healing. But after that Darshan, his focus became that of participation in the process of the disease, accepting it completely. Lance described this process during an interview at the Mountain Of Attention, where he and Robin were on retreat in September 1998. The interview was videotaped: Lance is seen sitting in his chair outside a retreat cabin. He is shirtless, his upper body and face tanned by the sun, his long black hair tied in a knot at the back of his head. Though paralyzed and wasted by Lou Gehrig's disease, one can still see the shadow of the once-healthy man. His face is mobile and full of life and humor. His voice, though altered by his illness, still has a hint of resonance, and he obviously enjoys talking.

LANCE: My first reaction to the disease was to not be present, to try and avoid feeling what was occurring. But by remaining in relationship with it, the process has become creative. Now it has become Spiritual practice.

Lance went on to say that the ability to practice beyond his fear, to stop seeking and demanding that life and consciousness continue in its present form, to accept rather than avoid and resist the change and transformation of death, was a Gift from his Divine Guru.

LANCE: It has become a tremendous opportunity to practice the relationship with Beloved Adi Da, to find out just how really true that is, how real it is.

He said that through his practice of devotional Remembrance and Invocation of Avatar Adi Da, he became increasingly able to feel his Divine Guru.

LANCE: The more you surrender your own subjectivity to Him, the less bound you are by all the variations, the physical pain and depression, the frustration that you can't do anything.

When asked by the interviewer to describe what it is like to "feel" Avatar Adi Da, Lance replied:

When I'm feeling Him most intensely I feel very happy, ridiculously so, like I have a bubble in my heart that just wants to laugh all the time. It's feeling happy without any reason. I mean, I have no reason to feel happy and yet <u>I feel</u> <u>happy</u>, sublime, really. I also feel very free but not in an ordinary way. I don't necessarily feel good [Lance smiles ruefully, casting his eyes down toward his body] either. It's more profound. I'm feeling beyond that. It's almost as if the "me", or the "I" of "me" is just a thought and not the reality. <u>He</u> is the Reality and <u>He</u> is arising as everything. <u>Happiness</u> is the Reality. Turning your attention to Him is not so much a relief but a rejoicing. It's Remembrance of the Eternal.

While Lance and Robin were in California that spring, they stayed with a longtime friend, Ian Morris, in the town of Graton in Sonoma County, about an hour's drive from the Mountain Of Attention Sanctuary. All three had observed how well Lance responded to the warmer weather in California, and Lance had even joked that maybe he could move into Ian's chicken coop out back. After his return to Canada, he began discussions with his network of friends in Graton (Zion, Robin's eldest son, also lived there) about the possibility of moving to California. He felt that he needed access to a larger community of devotees, to the Sanctuary, and to a more benign climate as his illness progressed. He asked his friends to help him die with dignity. Ian and Zion gathered their friends together for funding and building a small cabin on Ian's property.

In August, Lance, now in a wheelchair, moved to California and into his new little home, dubbing it "Last Face Chapel", a humorous combination of "Western Face Cathedral" and "Plain Talk Chapel", two temples named by Avatar Adi Da at the Mountain Of Attention.

After his move to Graton that summer, Lance got to know Ian and Zion's employers, Mimi and Peter Buckley, who live in Mill Valley. The Buckleys had been the owners of Esprit, a very successful clothing company. Mimi and Peter were touched by the plight of a young man dying of such a debilitating illness. Mimi saw that Lance was alone with "a bunch of guys", as she put it; and though they had the best of intentions, she felt they didn't have the experience or resources to care for someone as profoundly ill and disabled as Lance. She saw that he had special needs and that she and Peter had the means to provide for them.

Mimi was eager to help Lance for a number of reasons.

MIMI: He was really radiant, and he had such a great sense of humor, very devilish. He was like a homeopathic remedy for fear of death, because although he acknowledged the fear, it was not greater than the Divine Mystery he was surrendering into. His orientation to the Divine was so compelling and wonderful to be around. That quality of Divine Light illuminated him more and more as the process went on. It was tremendously healing. He let us into that experience and introduced us to Adi Da's Teaching. It was a great gift to us.

That summer and fall Lance spent more and more time down at the Buckleys' estate with a gathering of friends that steadily expanded to include nurses, bodyworkers, friends of Mimi's, and devotees of Avatar Adi Da.

MIMI: He created a family around him, and an extended community of caregiving was created by everybody's attraction to him.

Lance remarked in his interview on the graciousness of the Buckleys and how he felt Avatar Adi Da in everyone's loving service on his behalf.

◆ ◆ ◆

In late December of 1997, Lance's health took a dramatic turn for the worse. Feeling he might die soon, he wrote to Avatar Adi Da to tell Him so.

Avatar Adi Da responded by sending him His Love and Blessings, and an orange shawl (devotees wear special orange shawls on the Celebration of the Feast of the Horse-Sacrifice and in the death transition as a sign of renunciation) that He had put into the Sukra Kendra (a Temple reserved solely for use by Adi Da) for a few days. He also sent flower petals, sacred ash, and holy water, elements used in the daily, formal worship of Avatar Adi Da's

Murti. And He sent an audiotape with these Instructions: "No need for concern. Have no concerns. Practice My Teaching."

These Instructions were more fully elaborated in a Communication sent to Lance by Avatar Adi Da on January 17, 1998:

Send My Love and Blessings to Lance Barham. Tell him I am made fully aware of the situation, and read his letter. There is no need for concern. He should concentrate himself in the sadhana I have Given. Do that intensively, day to day. Practice this devotion to Me and forget "self".

These Instructions, Spoken directly to Lance from his Divine Heart-Master, carried great Blessing and purifying force. Immediately, Lance said humorously in the interview, he became incredibly concerned! He thought he was getting ready to die, and suddenly all the unhandled "concerns" that were buried in him came flooding to the surface; he became very busy arranging the details of his day-to-day life, so he could relinquish them. This "handling of business" was necessary, so that Lance's energy and attention could be free for the Spiritual process of ego-transcending Communion with Avatar Adi Da.

At this point, Mimi and Peter Buckley intervened again and decided that they would patronize Lance's medical needs entirely. He went to Stanford Medical Center in Palo Alto, California, where he received excellent treatment, and this reversed his rapid decline. His health stabilized, and he regained weight and strength. They also invited him to stay at their estate in Mill Valley as much as he wanted. As lovely as the cabin was in Graton, it was a small space and had none of the conveniences that made his life a bit easier. He accepted their offer.

LANCE: Mimi and Peter are extremely generous and gracious people. They provided me with financial support and offered me a place to stay that was exquisitely beautiful. Their place overlooks the city of San Francisco from near the top of Mt. Tamalpais. I was there six, seven hours a day in a state of mindless Communion with Beloved Adi Da. I had the sense that I was being held in His Huge Hands. I felt the world was in His Hands. It was sublime.

◆ ◆ ◆

"Do you want to go to Hawaii? You have five minutes to decide!"

It was February 1998, when Mimi hurried over to the house where Lance was staying with his friend Arthur Baker (the manager of the Buckleys' estate) and asked this question. Mimi and Peter were preparing to make a trip to Hawaii with their children. Mimi was looking out the window while making airplane reservations when she observed Lance out on the porch over at Arthur's, bundled up against the cold. It was the rainy California winter that accompanies the weather pattern of "El Nino", and they had not seen the sun for weeks. So, she thought, "Why not! Lance needs the sun." Lance and Mimi looked at one another in delight and disbelief. A few minutes later it was decided that Arthur, also a longtime devotee of Avatar Adi Da Samraj, would accompany Lance on his first trip to Hawaii. Lance quickly began to make arrangements for the two of them to go on a pilgrimage to Da Love-Ananda Mahal, an Adidam Retreat Sanctuary located on the island of Kauai.

"We flew to Hawaii first class," Lance said with delight, "and took a small plane to Kauai." They were greeted at Da Love-Ananda Mahal by William Tsiknas, a longtime devotee and resident of the Sanctuary, who showed them the different Holy Sites, temples and areas that had been infused with Avatar Adi Da's Spiritual Blessing, and told them stories of Avatar Adi Da's Divine Work there.

As they were preparing to leave, William paused for a moment, looked at them keenly, and said, "I had to meet you before telling you this, but Beloved Adi Da is on His way here. He'll be arriving tomorrow morning at 7:00 a.m., so come back in the morning at 6:45 and you can greet Him." Lance was flabbergasted.

LANCE: Being in Hawaii was a miracle, because Mimi's invitation to Kauai was out of the blue! Da Love-Ananda Mahal is so beautiful, so potent with Divine Power, and it was such a Grace just to be there. And then to find out that Adi Da was arriving and that we were invited to greet Him . . . [Lance shakes his head in disbelief] it was almost too much. It was just like "What is going on here"?

Arthur Baker tells the Leela of the next morning, in which various circumstances combined to delay their arrival, so that they weren't at the Sanctuary until 7:00 a.m.:

ARTHUR: Finally we get there. I throw open the doors of the car, set up the wheelchair, put Lance in the chair, and we charge up the hill. We join about twenty people in the driveway, and just as we settle into a position, Beloved Adi Da's car rolls in. The glass is tinted but we can see Him through it, and, unbelievably, He's looking right at Lance and me even before the door opens.

He steps out. He's wearing an indigo cotton suit in traditional Indian style and sandals, there are a couple of flower leis around His neck, offerings from devotees at the airport, and He's beaming this huge smile. His eyes are incredibly wide, and He looks around at everyone individually.

Then He looks at me and Lance and summons me forward with one simple gesture. Lance hasn't said anything. I wheel him right up to Beloved Adi Da, who is still standing by the open door of the car. Lance is close enough now for Beloved Adi Da to just reach out and place His hand directly on his head—which He does! As soon as His Hand touches Lance, there is this amazing column of Light. It was almost visible, but I could definitely feel it. It felt like Lance was ascending up this column and Beloved Adi Da's Descending Force was coming down. The love between them was just overwhelming. I could see the tears of Compassion in Beloved Adi Da's eyes, and the force of His Transmission was so intense His Hand was shaking a bit on top of Lance's head. The devotees behind us are weeping and exclaiming, praising Beloved Adi Da. He pulls His Hand back slightly, at which point everyone watching exhales for a moment. Then He strokes Lance's cheek with the back of His hand in the most tender of gestures. Finally, barely audibly, He Says the words "I Love you," and Lance says, "I love You."

At this point, I back up the wheelchair to give Beloved Adi Da room and He pauses to look around again at everyone. They are all praising and thanking Him. Lance and I are speechless. Beloved Adi Da is so vastly Present; His head seems to have grown to an impossible size, His eyes are so broad they almost seem to be working independently of one another, taking in everyone and every thing. Then Beloved Adi Da smiles a very sweet, small smile, picks up His Staff and, as William points out a few things regarding the new Temple, He goes into His House.

Later, Lance said that as soon as Avatar Adi Da touched his head he was enveloped in Light and overcome in a mindless, blissful swoon. He felt he was in a column of Light with immeasurable power. He said that he felt he could die now: he had never expected to see Avatar Adi Da again, and the Grace he had just received was incalculable. It was obvious to both Lance and Arthur that a great emotional and Spiritual healing was taking place for Lance.

LANCE: When He brushed my cheek with His Hand, I never felt love like that before, absolutely perfect, unlimited, unconditional love without any qualification. Nothing else could ever be so gracious.

And then Lance spoke of the end of the Prologue to *The Knee Of Listening,* which reads:

The Heart Is Real understanding. The Heart Is Real Consciousness and Real Life. The Heart Is What Merely and Only Is, but Which Is also Appearing In and Behind the conditions of mortal life and its death. Therefore, it is said of old, the One That Is Is neither born nor come to death, not Alive merely as the limitation of form (itself), not Itself (or Entirely) Rendered in what appears, and yet It Is the Living One, than Which there Is no lesser other (and no Great or Greater Other), Appearing As all of this Play of changes, but Eternally One, Unchanging, and Free.

There Is Only the Constant Knowledge and Enjoyment of the Heart, moment to moment, through the instant of all conditions of appearance and disappearance. Of This I Am Perfectly Certain. I Am That.

LANCE: I understood the Prologue in The Knee Of Listening *intuitively, perfectly. I saw Avatar Adi Da as Reality Itself, Eternal life, Deathless, Immortal, All-Pervading, Perfectly Free. I had felt that before with Beloved Adi Da, but in this instance it was tacit. I wasn't in the way so much. There was only Him. It was like He entered me and brushed me out. "You can go now, I'm taking over." [Lance laughs.] I felt free, free in an ecstatic way. That sense has stayed with me. He removed a lot that was in the way of feeling Him.*

Lance returned to California. He did not expect to live beyond a few more months or see his Beloved Adi Da again.

LANCE: I went back to Mill Valley, and my friends and patrons knew that I needed to have my Spiritual practice available to me, so a Murti of Beloved Adi Da was installed. There were several months of joyous celebration there with family and friends. Beloved Adi Da was very present, and you could feel Him dominating the atmosphere. People were always commenting, "Why is it so happy here? Why does it feel so good? Why is this guy so alive when he's dying?" It had nothing to do with me. I kept telling everyone it's my Guru, that's what He does, that's what He is.

That April, on his 39th birthday, Lance sent Beloved Adi Da a card with a frog on it. A big birthday party was arranged and Lance had an altar prepared and the Murti set up for the occasion. That evening he noticed a live frog sitting on the altar next to the Murti and pointed it out to his friends.

LANCE: Everybody was amazed, because no one had seen a frog up there in years. All of a sudden you could feel Beloved Adi Da so intensely. His Descent was palpable and people went wild with ecstasy. Most had no idea why.

AVATAR ADI DA SAMRAJ: Death requires a loving, fearless, sorrowless, unangered volunteer of me. Death requires the feeling heart's participation—enamored, self-forgetting, and without anticipation. [The Mummery]

In early July, Avatar Adi Da traveled to the Mountain Of Attention. Now living again in Graton, Lance and Robin traveled to the Sanctuary to participate in the devotional culture on weekends. On the morning of July 26, Avatar Adi Da asked about whether or not Lance would be at the Sanctuary that day. Avatar Adi Da was told that he would be—and He then suggested that Lance and Robin stay at one of the retreat cabins on the Sanctuary. And so began the last four months of Lance Barham's life, where he would be Gracefully drawn beyond himself into being a "loving, fearless, sorrowless, unangered volunteer".

Lance remarked on how Graceful it was for Avatar Adi Da to Invite him to stay on retreat at the Mountain Of Attention for as long it was medically prudent and Lance was physically able to do so.

LANCE: He gave me the great gift to let my life go here on this Holy land. It's nothing I could have thought up or wished for on my own. To be here, to live on the Sanctuary, to see Beloved Adi Da all the time, to die in the Company of my Guru? No, I could never have dreamt this up.

That same day, there was also an occasion in which Avatar Adi Da Sat formally in Darshan with many devotees. At the end of the Darshan, Avatar Adi Da rose from His Seat and walked to the side of the room where Lance was sitting in his wheelchair. He stood in front of Lance, His Face radiant with Compassion, tears falling from His Eyes. He put His Hand on Lance's forehead, keeping it there for about a minute. Many in the room were weeping, heart-penetrated by the sight of the Divine Person's death-overwhelming Love, a Love that is with everyone at all times, in life, at death, after death, Eternally.

After this occasion, Lance wrote a letter to Avatar Adi Da.

My Adi Da,

Thank You so, so much! You are Absolute Love-Bliss. You have Said "Everything has already died, this is the other world". This is what I felt today with Your Darshan. I felt the Great Tree from Hridaya Rosary, and my head melted away. I felt so Free in Bliss and so in Love with You.

When you pressed the ajna point on my forehead I felt perfectly penetrated, like a hole. I don't even know who I am, nor do I care. I am so happy to see You. You are so Sublime and so Beautiful.

During Darshan, I had a vision of the Cosmic Mandala. It looked like a tunnel with You as the Divine Star. It was huge. The Mandala was all I could see, with You in the Center. My primary feeling was that I felt like I had already died and that I was Entirely with You.

The whole world should be bowing at Your Feet.

So much happened that I couldn't put it all into words and yet nothing was going on. Just You! You are the only One. It is true there is Only You!

Your tears on my legs felt like the light of diamonds, and they penetrated every cell in my body with "Brightness". I am so happy to be here. I'll do what I can to serve You by bringing devotees to You. I do not know if I have much time though, but whatever time I have I will be shouting Your Name loud and far. I am so grateful for being here at the Mountain Of Attention. Thank You for Inviting me here.

Your eternal devotee,
Lance

Hridaya Rosary

Lance's letter includes many references to *Hridaya Rosary,* one of Avatar Adi Da's "Source-Texts" that describes the "Healing Pose", or the process of letting Adi Da's Spiritual Blessing, Which is Infinitely above the body-mind, "Melt" the entire being, including the "Great Tree" of subtle existence that rises above the "root-ball" of the brain. Lance also talks about the "ajna" point, a point of Spiritual contact on the forehead just above and between the eyes. And he tells Adi Da that he had a vision of the "Cosmic Mandala", the multi-colored circle of cosmic Light that has at its center Avatar Adi Da in His Divine Five-Pointed Star-Form.

AVATAR ADI DA SAMRAJ: In the Yoga of devotion to Me, you do not "come up" to Me. Rather, you allow the Melting that permits Me to Descend to you. That allowing of the Melting is self-surrender and self-forgetting. Therefore, the paradox of the Spiritual Process in My Avataric Divine Heart-Company is that, in your reception of Me, "you" are gone, forgotten. You are simply an openness, without egoic self-reference. [Hridaya Rosary]

Throughout that summer and fall, Adi Da Samraj Graced His devotees with many occasions of Darshan. Lance participated in all these events, which were resonantly sublime with the Promised God-Man's Transmission of His Love-Bliss. Avatar Adi Da kept abreast of Lance's physical condition through the community's doctors. And He clarified for Lance—and for all His devotees—what the practice of self-yielding and self-forgetting should be in Adidam when facing physical death:

AVATAR ADI DA SAMRAJ: Lance's practice at this point should be profound and not superficial. He is obviously in the last stages of his life, and, as I have recommended, My devotees who are in this process should go on retreat instead of trying to perpetuate the conventions of life in the ordinary sense. He has to adapt to the most profound devotional resort, and this involves a heart-opening to Me from head to toe. Certainly, it involves the head opening from the heart. Whatever stage of practice an individual is in, this is fundamental to the death process. In death, all that is below the head disappears, so there is no more "head to toe" about it—there is just everything above the head. It is possible in life for practice to become so profound that at times there is no physical awareness and just heart-Communion with Me, an awareness of everything above and beyond the body and the fullness of the total Sphere of My Form without any particular physical pattern.

He should have significant time for solitary practice. He should have someone near him in case he needs anything, but those serving him should be on retreat and in a unique disposition. It is not about keeping up with appearances of social personality or social existence. All of that should be relaxed more and more. Heart-Communion with Me should be the mode of life in these last stages.

Lance, through devotion to his Divine Guru, was being drawn more and more deeply into feeling beyond himself to the All-Pervading Divine Body and "Bright" Transcendental Person of Avatar Adi Da Samraj. But Lance said it was not he, Lance, who was somehow "achieving" this Spiritual depth. Through the miracle of Avatar Da's Grace, Lance was able to feel beyond his egoic inclinations of fear, sorrow, and anger.

LANCE: Beloved Adi Da is Outshining that. It arises, but it has so little force in me. It's not as if I'm really doing anything. I'm not effortfully practicing the Way of Adidam. It is about Remembering Beloved Adi Da, Communing with Him prior to all that. He is doing it. What I see is that He Loves His devotees. He Loves them absolutely and perfectly. I don't deserve all of this and it really has nothing to do with me personally. It has to do with Love, with Who He Is, and I am so grateful. I hope to see Him a few more times. I am getting weaker now, and soon it will be time to go.

By early November it was clear that it would soon be time for Lance to leave the Sanctuary. He had stopped eating and was taking only water. He had become too weak to sit in Darshan. He was beginning the process of letting the body go. He saw his Beloved Adi Da for the last time at a Darshan occasion at Seventh Gate, a Holy Site at the Sanctuary, and then it was time to go. Avatar Adi Da had been informed that Lance would be leaving the Sanctuary on November 12, and He had Said that Lance should continue to communicate with Him. He wanted to be assured that Lance's personal care had been properly arranged, and He sent His Love and Blessings.

It was about three in the afternoon on a beautiful day, with the winter sun spreading its pale, golden light over the Sanctuary, when Lance and Robin began the drive back to Graton. It was heart-breaking for Robin, who knew this would be their last ride together. As they left the Sanctuary, an eagle—quite rare in the area—suddenly appeared and flew alongside the car. They slowed to watch as it alighted on a fence post. It seemed a powerful sign to them, in keeping with Lance's Native American heritage, a sign of blessing and of farewell.

Lance died on the morning of Wednesday, November 18. He spent the night before his death with his friends and family. They read to him from the Wisdom-Teaching of Avatar Adi Da, and laughed with him about old times. Lance communicated his love for everyone that night.

Mary Graham, a devotee living in the area, and a member of Mate Moce, was with Lance in the late evening. Lance told her that he was fading in and out, and that it was "Bright". He said. "I'm going to the 'Bright'". He wanted to say more, so she came to sit by his side. His breathing was labored, and he was whispering.

Lance told her that he had asked Beloved Adi Da about the practice in death and had received the Instruction: "Feel Me Infinitely Above and shoot straight to Me like an arrow." Lance said that he had seen how Avatar Adi Da does the whole process of the ego-forgetting, ego-transcending Way of Adidam from "inside us", dissolving the ego until we are not there anymore. "But then you don't need to be there," he said. "You're not needed, and Beloved Adi Da just continues to do His Work once we are out of the way." He and Mary laughed together in recognition of this Divine Happiness and Freedom from "self".

Lance was radiant as he communicated the pleasure of his surrender, of his being "Outshined" by the Divine Person. He talked about how with Beloved Adi Da's Birth, the Divine has been Revealed as the Truth of life. He said, "Before Beloved Adi Da, this was never the case. Now it is. It's going to take some time to incarnate this great Revelation, to introduce a new world religion. We will be here for lifetimes of practice. What a happy thought, this practice! Beloved Adi Da has made it clear what it is we have to do: Invoke Him here. The practice is about no more un-Happiness. In Darshan, Beloved Adi Da Reveals His Sign, He Reveals that He Is Who, and who we Are. There is no 'difference'. It's amazing. There is no where to go!"

Adi Da Samraj Writes in *The Mummery*:

To die is necessary, in Life's poor Mummery—but, it is not Right and True, unless it is enacted from the feeling-heart. To die by yielding bodily, from the feeling-heart—as when in the Embrace of body-love—is <u>perfect</u> trust, beyond every thought of the little bed of "I"-and-"other"-in-a-room. Such feeling-death exceeds <u>all</u> loss of human love—by means of the human heart's felt constant Un-denial of the Divine Inherent Fullness of Reality's own Love-Bliss.

Avatar Adi Da received word of Lance's passing on the morning of November 18, 1998.

◆ ◆ ◆

Bodily death is not an "end" to life but a change, a transition. And that transition—the relinquishment of association with the body-mind—usually takes about three days. In Adidam, devotees conduct a three-day, around-the-clock vigil for a person who has died—three days of prayer, puja, chants, and recitations of Avatar Adi Da's Wisdom-Teaching to help the practitioner make his or her transition in the context of surrender into the Heart of the Divine Person. And everyone who participates is aided in his or her right understanding of death, is healed at depth by the Love-Blissful Presence of the Divine Person and is helped in the process of mutual release.

For the vigil, Lance's body was placed in a coffin that a devotee had built for him, and the orange shawl of renunciation that Avatar Adi Da had Given to him was wrapped around his shoulders. Over the next three days, the little house he had so humorously called "Last Face Chapel" became a Temple that was potent with Avatar Adi Da's Love-Blissful Descent. As friends, family, and devotees entered to participate in the vigil many remarked on how it felt as if they were entering to receive Avatar Adi Da's Darshan. By the second day, most devotees felt that Lance was separated from his physical body, and that the vigil had become a celebration of worship of the Divine.

The last day of the vigil ended in an ecstatic celebration, which began with a puja on Avatar Adi Da's Murti, followed by sacred music and chanting led by one of Avatar Adi Da's daughters, Trivedi Tamarind Free Jones. The little cottage was jammed with people singing at the top of their lungs, while the pungent smell of burning sage filled the room (a request by Lance to honor his Native American heritage).

Mimi and Peter Buckley came with their children, who, says Mimi, took to the scene's contagious, high energy. Mimi felt it was illuminating to see everyone's faces so full of light and happiness. Her children all left flowers in Lance's coffin, and her youngest child remarked later on how beautiful Lance had looked.

MIMI: Lance had this characteristic little humorous smile on his face. But I could see that what had been a home was now like a shell on the beach. It was possible to say good-bye. It was an incredibly healing event. It was healing in every single way.

Lance had his last joke when it came time to take the coffin to the crematorium. Everyone tumbled out of the cottage chanting ecstatically while the hearse drivers looked on, wide-eyed. Suddenly everything came to a halt; Arthur and Zion, who were carrying the coffin, couldn't get it through the door. They looked at one another, took the lid off, turned him sideways and went through the narrow door that way. As one person remarked, "It was so perfectly Lance."

◆ ◆ ◆

One month later, Avatar Adi Da Samraj was in conversation with a group of His devotees, "considering" the nature of Reality.

AVATAR ADI DA SAMRAJ: Now, today what is the status of Lance? What is the status of you in your knowing of anyone? The only difference between Lance today and Lance a few weeks ago is the introduction of Consciousness in association with a pile of material that got named Lance. Where do you have to go to name it now? That pile of matter fell into a pile of dust and blew away. It's a zillion other things now. So it seems like Reality Is What Is Being the Case and not Lance. Or when it seemed there was a Lance, it wasn't Lance that was Being the Case. It was Reality Being the Case. And now, when you are having your turn at seeming to be the case, it is not you that is Being the Case at all! Reality is Being the Case! And there isn't "anyone" about it at all. The pattern is changing, but it isn't being any "one" or "thing" but only Itself at any time. Reality is Being the Case whether you are the case or not. Any apparent "anything" or apparent "anyone" coincides inherently, Perfectly with the Only One.

This Leela of Avatar Adi Da's Avataric Divine Grace Outshining the mortal point-of-view is not just a lesson about how to live the final years or days of our lives; it is a lesson for today. Truthfully, we are all, even now, in Lance's situation. The threat of death only highlights the temporality of the dream that is the body-mind, the "I". Lance, because of his terminal illness, was no longer as beguiled by that dream. There was almost nothing to distract him from mortality, and his need for heart-surrender to the Divine Person. By Means of the Avataric Divine Grace of His Divine Heart-Master, he was profoundly deepened in that practice of surrender, which transcends the illusions of "I". As Avatar Adi Da Samraj Writes about the True "I", or Personhood:

AVATAR ADI DA SAMRAJ: Your True Personhood is Immeasurably Beyond your egoically "personal" bodily (human) form. Your "personal" (or egoically separated) bodily (human) form is only a transparent (or merely apparent), and un-necessary, and inherently non-binding modification of Me, the One and Only and Very Divine (or Eternal, Great, and Inherently egoless) Person. [Aham Da Asmi (Beloved, I Am Da)]

May all of us be Blessed to transcend the mortal "I" in the "Bright" Heart of Reality, Happiness Itself, the Great egoless Person of the Ruchira Avatar, Adi Da Samraj.

PART FIVE

Children and Death

This part of the guide focuses on concerns specific to the death of a child or a child's loved-one. This instruction is compiled from the experience of Mate Moce.

How to Serve a Child Who Is Dying

It is best to serve young practitioners of the Way of Adidam who are dying by helping them resort to the same practices they have used in life. Use the same prayers and language that they are familiar with, such as the exercises for looking, feeling, and being more than what we look like. (You can refer to booklet 3 of the "Conscious Childrearing" booklet series, *The Practice of Ecstasy with Children.*) Help them resort to Avatar Adi Da through saying His Name, mala-japa, etc. All of these practices should be engaged and intensified with young practitioners who are dying. This is essentially His same Instruction to adults also. Avatar Adi Da Asks us to deepen our surrender to Him and our devotional resort to Him. Devotional music and soft chanting may be an important and useful thing to enjoy together. Instructions in simple breathing and "conductivity" exercises regarding letting go of the physical body in an upward direction would also be useful in preparation for death and as death approaches.

In reading instructions at the time of death, you would use the age of the child and his or her comprehension of Avatar Adi Da's Wisdom-Teaching as a guide. You could adapt Avatar Adi Da's Instructions for younger children and tell them to "feel through everything arising to the feeling of the Mystery, or the feeling of Beloved Adi Da . . .", and so on.

Here is an example of how you might read Avatar Adi Da's Instructions for young people (adapted by Molly Jones in her book *The Sky Goes On Forever*):

You might see a bright white star. It is good to look right at this star for as long as you can when you see it, and let yourself go up toward it.

Let go of everything and look or feel up and to the center of where you are now, and let yourself go up. Look or feel toward God, or Love, or the Spirit, or the bright white light, or the bright white star. They are all the same thing. Feel the Spirit. Stay in the Spirit. Rest in the Spirit. You will know that it is the Spirit because it will feel like Love.

Practitioners have asked us whether it is necessary to do a full three-day vigil for an infant. Avatar Adi Da Samraj has Said that a very young infant or a fetus lost in the womb has hardly any awareness of the physical body, so that the death and transition processes occur quickly and rather simultaneously. He has Said there is no reason to engage a full three-day vigil or to do verbal prayers and chanting.

Because the infant had not yet begun the process of engaging the verbal mind, the service should be a simple feeling and releasing process, done mostly for the adults, who must now release all their attachment and sorrow regarding the infant. The vigil should be engaged for a long enough period of time to encourage the parents' and family's release in all the same ways we do with an older individual's passing.

The older the child is, the more verbally and bodily aware he or she has become. Thus, an older dying child should be served much as we would serve an adult. He or she should be helped to release all attachments to parents, family, pets, and possessions and to relax all fear about the death process.

How to Serve Children Who Are Grieving

Death is happening around us all the time. It is important to introduce children to death through ordinary everyday instances. Natural occasions to discuss death would include the death of plants in fall and winter or if one finds a dead bird or other creature while on a walk. Death of a pet can provide a very real opportunity for a child, not only to learn about death, but to learn to handle the feelings of loss. It is important for children to encounter these feelings before having to deal with the loss of a person they love.

A child's comprehension of death varies with age. Understanding the finality of death of the body is dependent partly on the child's stage of cognitive development. Generally, preschool children see death as reversible, temporary, and impersonal. The finality of death is denied. Child psychology books tell us that between ages five and nine death is seen to exist, but it can be avoided (only <u>some</u> people die). Children in this age group often harbor the idea that somehow they can escape death through their ingenuity and efforts. At about age nine or ten, death is understood to be an inevitable occurrence that happens to all people. Some children may comprehend death quite a bit earlier, especially children who are dying themselves.

Children should be helped to understand the difference between life and death. If they bury a dead bird, they may worry that the bird will get cold and lonely or get hungry and not be able to breathe under the dirt. Explain to them that the bird's body no longer thinks, breathes, or feels. The body dies and will not revive. But, according to Beloved Adi Da, it can be explained that just as "You and I are more than what we look like", the bird is also more than what it looks like. The bird continues to live in the Mystery.

Avatar Adi Da Samraj explains death to children:

> *Some day, everybody has what they look like go to sleep and not wake up. Then they forget that part, and they go on to someplace else and look different. Nobody knows what they will look like after what they look like now goes to sleep forever. When you go to sleep at night, you forget what you looked like all day. And when somebody dies, or lets the body go to sleep for the last time, they forget what they looked like when they were alive and awake. It is a Mystery—like going to sleep, or dreaming, or waking up.*
>
> *. . . you are always <u>more</u> than what you <u>look</u> like. The part that is the way you look is only you while you are awake and alive. But the rest of you goes on while you sleep and dream—and, after the body dies (or goes to sleep for good), the rest of you goes on in the Mystery.*
> [What, Where, When, How, Why, and <u>Who</u> To Remember To Be Happy]

When a loved one, parent, sibling, grandparent, or friend is dying, children should be informed. Children of all ages should be allowed to visit and to be involved in caring for a dying person with whom they are intimate. When death actually occurs, children should be told clearly and directly what has happened. It isn't helpful to tell a child that the person has simply "gone away" or that "God has taken the person to be with Him", since this can be misleading and confusing. The death of the body is real, and children must be told that they will not be seeing their loved one's body any more. But it is also an opportunity to rediscover and discuss with a child that everyone is more than what they look like, and therefore the death of the physical body is a part of the Mystery.

Telling young children that sickness was the cause of death can also create problems, if the truth is not tempered with reassurance. Preschoolers cannot differentiate between temporary and fatal illness, and minor ailments may begin to cause them unnecessary concern. When talking to a child about someone who has died as a result of illness, it might be helpful to explain that only a very serious illness may cause death, and that although we all get sick sometimes, we usually get better again.

As you are talking to a child about death, be sensitive to the child's concerns and use words that he/she understands. In his book *Talking about Death: A Dialogue Between Parent and Child*, Earl Grollman tells a humorous story. "Children often mistake the meanings of words and phrases. I was once asked by a young girl, 'How long is death?' I responded, 'Death is permanent.' The youngster said, 'Oh, then it's not so bad.' Noticing my bewilderment she said simply, 'My mother has permanents all the time. It lasts for about six months.'"[1]

When young children are informed of a loved one's serious illness or death, psychologists report their behavior frequently changes for a period of time. They may become more dependent or submissive or deny what they are feeling.

Children should be encouraged to express whatever they are feeling. They will feel greater freedom to do this if their parents (and other adults around them) freely express themselves in their presence rather than trying to hide their grief. This gives the child permission to do the same.

A young child may not be able to talk directly about death. In conventional society, art and therapeutic play have been effective ways for small children to communicate about death and grief. In Adidam, puja, sacred occasion, and truly sacred art would be our best means of resorting to Avatar Adi Da and allowing for the release of grieving emotions.

When a child experiences the death of a close relative, they often feel guilty. While most of us experience some guilt when losing a loved one, young children, in particular, have difficulty understanding cause and effect relationships. They often think that in some way they caused the death. Maybe their angry thoughts caused the person to die. Children may need help coping with guilt by asking about their concerns and receiving reassurance that they have always been loved and still are. It may also help to explain the circumstances of the death.

The death of a close relative also arouses feelings of anger in children. Children are apt to express their angry feelings openly, especially when they've lost someone on whom they depended for love and care. Adults need to accept children's feelings and reassure children that they will be cared for. Children should be helped to cope with feelings of loss in the way Avatar Adi Da has Instructed young people to handle any feelings. He Says in *What, Where, When, How, Why, and <u>Who</u> To Remember To Be Happy*:

> *If you will remember every day to feel and breathe the Mystery, and if you will remember to feel that you are more than what you look like, and if you will remember to <u>Be</u> the Mystery Itself—then you will be happy every day. . . .*

1. Grollman, Earl A., *Talking about Death: A Dialogue Between Parent and Child* (Boston, Mass.: Beacon Press, 1970), p. xii.

Remembering the Mystery is a way of being everything you always already are. When you sleep, you are something different than when you wake up. And when you dream, you are different, too. The way you seem to be when you wake up is only one of the ways you are.

Just keep on remembering that you, with everybody else, do not know what even a single thing Is. . . .

As practitioners of Adidam, it is our practice, and the practice of our children, to go beyond the body every day, to know that we are more than what we look like. In doing this, we are preparing for death every day.

If a child is to visit a dying relative in a hospital or attend a funeral or vigil, he or she should be prepared ahead of time for what to expect. Tell the child how the person or body may look, what the room will be like, etc. Remind the child to bring good energy to the occasion. Provide an opportunity afterward for the child to discuss his or her feelings with an adult.

If a child who has lost an intimate persists in having fears of death, expresses a desire to die in order to be with the dead parent or other intimate, has frequent outbursts of anger and seems to feel guilty, attempts to take care of a surviving parent, seems unable to express his or her feelings and/or seems suddenly lethargic, extra help (perhaps including professional help) may be required to help the child cope with the loss.

A properly handled death and vigil will certainly help minimize fixation in grief for both children and adults. The vigil should be a positive devotional occasion with the constant emphasis on feeling-Contemplation of Avatar Adi Da Samraj, and releasing attachment to the one who has died.

A Leela of a Child's Death

Told by Shawn Lipscomb

The following Leela is an excellent example of helping children through the death of an intimate. It is told by devotee Shawn Lipscomb, a teacher who runs a private school in Lake County, California. In 1994, Justino, a preschooler in Shawn's school, died. After being found unconscious, he was revived and kept on life-support for about a week before he finally died. Because the cause of his death was unknown, an autopsy was ordered. Devotees serving Justino were unable to prevent the autopsy, but were at least able to have it delayed for several hours. After the autopsy, the boy's body was returned and a vigil was performed at that time.

Justino's older sister, Kristina, was in Shawn's kindergarten class at the time. Shawn tells the story of how the children in the preschool and kindergarten classes were served during Justino's death and also how they served Justino and Kristina.

I was one of the people who was at the hospital with Justino, both before his death and directly afterwards. Before I went down to the hospital to serve him, I was almost dreading it, thinking it was going to be really hard. I was also afraid that, because I was so closely associated with Justino, I would be overcome with emotion and unable to serve. I found, though, that in serving him, I was served myself. Particularly in doing the readings from *What, Where, When, How, Why, and Who To Remember To Be Happy*, I became ecstatic. And so did everyone else who was around Justino. What I had envisioned as a grim, awful circumstance wasn't that way at all. Everyone who was serving him felt a lot of love. It was really a very positive and strong event.

The nurses and the doctors were also very moved by hearing *What, Where, When, How, Why, and Who To Remember To Be Happy* read, and by the way everything was served in a very life-positive way. They were extremely respectful and helpful in whatever ways they could be. They were impressed that there is actually a way to serve a death, and it didn't have to be so grim. (This was in the children's intensive care unit where they have children dying all the time.) They wanted to know more about Beloved Adi Da, His Wisdom-Teaching, and the Way of Adidam.

The day after Justino died was a school day. The preschool teacher and I got all the kids together in the preschool and kindergarten classes. We talked to them about what had happened, explaining that Justino had gone to sleep in the Mystery. Then we read the story of *Badger's Parting Gifts*, which is a children's book about grief. Badger's parting gifts are all the things that he had taught his friends before he died. He taught Mole to cut out a chain of moles from folded paper. He taught Frog to skate, Fox to tie his tie, and Mrs. Rabbit to make gingerbread rabbits. When the animals recount his gifts, they feel connected to Badger and happy. Thus, the story instructs children about finding a continuing, living connection with someone who has died.

We talked about finding our living connection with Justino, even though he was going through a change and we wouldn't see his body anymore. Some of the kids remembered songs that he liked. One remembered that he liked miner's grass and would pick a lot of it in the springtime. So the children said they would remember Justino when they picked miner's grass.

We also talked about animals or other intimates who had died, and the children shared any experiences that they had had. And we read Molly Jones's book, *The Sky Goes On Forever*, together.

Next we talked about the vigil that would be occurring. We told the children that Justino was being brought to a friend's house, and that we could go there to see him and say goodbye. I told them what he would probably look like. He would be pale looking, and his body would be cold and he wouldn't be breathing. I also talked about how they did an operation after he was dead (the autopsy), to find out why he died, and told the children they might see some stitches in his hair. (I emphasized that it didn't hurt because he was already dead.) I told the children that he would still look like Justino, and they might also be able to feel him and recognize him that way.

We talked about what we would like to bring him, what kind of energy we could give and what we could do. Some of the children wanted to say a prayer to him, and others wanted to sing to him. So we talked about what songs we could sing. They decided to sing one of the songs they had recently learned about breathing and feeling the Mystery, and being happy in the Mystery. Justino had particularly liked that song. They also chose to sing the Brahms Lullaby, which they had recently learned. They felt like it was something that would help Justino go to sleep in the Mystery.

The next day after school, we went over to the vigil with the preschoolers and kindergartners. (This was all done with the parents' permission.) Kristina was going to meet the classes there. This would be the first time the children had seen Kristina since Justino's death. We talked with the children about how it would help her to have her friends there with her. I specifically noticed that all the children were completely fine about what was happening.

The children all had flowers to offer. We went over to the vigil house and waited in the living room for Kristina to join us. When Kristina arrived, the children all gave her hugs and were happy to see her. We all got ready to go in to the vigil room together. The children got their flowers, and we talked about walking in quietly, so as not to disturb what was going on. We explained to the children who were not devotees of Beloved Adi Da that there would be a picture of Justino's and Kristina's Spiritual Teacher in the room. We also described how Justino would be in a box on the floor with a sheet up to his chest. They would be able to see his face. We told them it would be best not to disturb the body, such as pulling down the sheet. They asked if they could touch him, and we said, "Yes, you can touch him gently on his face or on his hair." We also said that they could put their flowers in the box with him, as well as at the picture of Beloved Adi Da.

We went in and sat with Justino's body, and the children sang their songs and said prayers. All the children touched him, and stroked his hair and the side of his face. They were all very sensitive and calm. A couple of the kids went around to the other side of the box to look for his stitches. We all sat quietly for a little while. Just before it was time to go, a few of the children said goodbye and told him to be happy in the Mystery. Then we went out.

None of the kids seemed disturbed in the least. They acted like it was completely ordinary and natural, and the right thing to do.

What was so impressive to me was that the kids didn't seem to have any natural fear of death. I saw that if adults allow children to participate in the death process, it becomes what it really is—a natural part of all of life. For them, there was nothing strange or negative about it. Even seeing a dead body was completely fine with them. None of the kids held back. They all touched Justino and talked to him and were completely at ease.

Even afterwards, they talked amongst themselves about how he looked, and how his body was cold. But there was nothing creepy or morbid about it. I don't remember any of them getting particularly sorrowful or strange with it, either. And they didn't seem to be avoiding it. It was completely happy and fine to them.

In the weeks following, the children continued to talk about Justino's death, and it seemed like a completely ordinary, but also very feeling conversation. When Kristina came back to school, the children were able to help her with her grief whenever it would arise. They would come to her side, remind her that Justino was in the Mystery, and help her breathe in the good stuff and breathe out the bad stuff.

(NOTE: Singing familiar songs and touching the face of the person who has died are not recommended for adults, but did seem to help the children learn about and accept their friend's death. After children or a non-devotee family member has been with the body, the devotees attending the vigil should intensify their efforts to help the deceased to release, perhaps by waving lights and incense, giving verbal instructions and telling the one who has died that the family member will be all right without them.)

PART SIX

Readings

During the death transition, people's experience can be very chaotic, especially shortly after physical death. Therefore, instructions to such individuals need to be simple and clear. Reading an entire Essay from *Easy Death* will probably not be very useful for one who has died. However, it is often useful during a vigil for the individuals serving the vigil to read some of these Essays to help align themselves to Beloved Adi Da's Wisdom about death.

Any of the following excerpts and Essays would be helpful for a devotee who is approaching death to serve his or her preparation for the death transition.

Also, see the section on formal recitations during the three-day vigil (p. 52) for how best to use these readings in a vigil.

Recommended Readings from Avatar Adi Da's Wisdom-Teaching

"My Divine Disclosure," printed in each of the Twenty-Three "Source-Texts"

Readings from *Easy Death*

* Chapters 24 and 25 about the Cosmic Mandala
* Chapter 38, "Death Is a Living Process"
* Chapters 40, 41, and 42 on Grief
* "What Is Wonderful Is Not Threatened", p. 82
* "Death Is a Perfect Insult", p. 257

Readings for Children

* The "Conscious Childrearing" booklet series, published by the Vision of Mulund Institute (available from the Adidam Emporium)
* *The Fall of Freddie the Leaf*, by Leo Buscaglia (Thorofare, N.J.: Charles B. Slack, 1982) (a children's book about death)
* *Badger's Parting Gifts*, by Susan Varley (New York: Morrow & Company, First Mulberry Edition, 1992)
(a children's book about grieving)

Attached Readings from Avatar Adi Da's Wisdom-Teaching (starting on p. 97)

* *Da Love-Ananda Gita*, verses 49 and 50
* Prologue from *The Knee Of Listening*
* "The Secret, or Law, of the Death Process"
* "The Vision of Eternal Life"
* "Only Life Overcomes Death"
* "Original Light"
* Epilogue from *Ishta*

Attached Readings from Avatar Adi Da's Wisdom-Teaching—

Da Love-Ananda Gita

verses 49 and 50

49.

Do not Meditate on your separate self (your states, your experiences, your presumed knowledge, your dilemma, your problem, or your search), and do not perpetuate self-contraction (by strategies of independent effort, and by adventures of either self-glorification or self-destruction, within or without)—but (always, immediately) transcend self-Meditation, personal states, conditional experiences, presumptions of knowledge, and all of dilemma, problem, and search (Merely by Remembering Me, and Invoking Me, and heart-Recognizing Me, and Meditating on Me, and, Therefore, Merely by surrendering to Me—not by self-concerned effort, or by isolated and concerned manipulation of conditions themselves, but by simply, and intentionally, and more and more deeply, responding and Yielding to the always presently Available feeling of the Inherent "Bright" Attractiveness of My Avatarically-Born bodily human Divine Form, and of My Avatarically Self-Revealed Spiritual, and Always Blessing, Divine Presence, and of My Avatarically Self-Revealed, and Very, and Transcendental, and Perfectly Subjective, and Inherently Spiritual, and Inherently egoless, and Inherently Perfect, and Self-Evidently Divine State), and (Thus, by Means of the always presently Available Grace That Is My Good Company) always and actively feel beyond and (really, effectively) transcend your separate and separative self (Merely by feeling, and Thereby Contemplating, Me).

50.

Do this Contemplation for Its own Sake, and not passively and partially (as if waiting for devotion to happen to you, rather than always presently Remembering, Invoking, and heart-Recognizing Me, and, Thereupon, responsively allowing the presently inevitable feeling of My Inherent "Bright" Attractiveness, and, Thereby, most simply, always and fully activating My always Given and Giving Gift of devotion), and not cleverly and strategically (with all effort and no heart-response, intent but not Yielding, stressful with the seeking of Me, rather than Happy with the Finding of Me)—but do this Contemplation constantly, always, Merely, and by heart, and (Thus) by feeling to My Avatarically-Born bodily (human) Divine Form, and by feeling into My Avatarically Self-Revealed Spiritual (and Always Blessing) Divine Presence, and (more and more) by feeling My Very and Freely Avatarically-Self-Revealed and Freely (Inherently) Perfect State.

[For further reading from the *Da Love-Ananda Gita*, see verses 1-52 and 90-108.]

The Heart of Understanding

Prologue to *The Knee Of Listening*

Death is utterly acceptable to consciousness and life. There has been endless time of numberless deaths, but neither consciousness nor life has ceased to arise. The felt quality and cycle to death has not modified the fragility of flowers, even the flowers within the human body. Therefore, one's understanding of consciousness and life must be turned to That Utter, Inclusive Truth, That Clarity and Wisdom, That Power and Untouchable Gracefulness, That One and Only Reality, this evidence suggests. One must cease to live in a superficial and divided way, seeking and demanding consciousness and life in the present apparent form, avoiding and resisting what appears to be the end of consciousness and life in death.

The Heart Is Real understanding. The Heart Is Real Consciousness and Real Life. The Heart Is What Merely and Only Is, but Which Is also Appearing In and Behind the conditions of mortal life and its death. Therefore, it is said of old, the One That Is Is neither born nor come to death, not Alive merely as the limitation of form (itself), not Itself (or Entirely) Rendered in what appears, and yet It Is the Living One, than Which there Is no lesser other (and no Great or Greater Other), Appearing As all of this Play of changes, but Eternally One, Unchanging, and Free.

There Is Only the Constant Knowledge and Enjoyment of the Heart, moment to moment, through the instant of all conditions of appearance and disappearance. Of This I Am Perfectly Certain. I Am That.

The Secret, or Law, of the Death Process

May 21, 1980

The "secret", or Law, of the death process is the same that applies to the existence during your born lifetime: The right relationship to the process is that of love-surrender, not recoil or withdrawal. The death process is simply another form of participation in the Mystery and Universal Unity of existence. Death is not self-suppression. It is not a process whereby the "self" is reduced to zero or thrown into eternal chaos. Such a passage, if it seems to arise, either during your lifetime or in the process of death, is a hallucination created by your own recoiling fear. In any case, the hallucination eventually vanishes, and it will vanish most quickly and permanently if you will surrender the egoic self through feeling into Ecstatic Love-Communion with Me—the Avatarically Self-Revealed Transcendental, Inherently Spiritual, and Self-Evidently Divine Self-Condition (and Source-Condition) of All and all.

The death process should not be engaged merely as a retreat from embodiment. It should not be used to retreat <u>into</u> the "self". Rather, it should be engaged as self-surrender, or love-surrender of the total body-mind. As when going to sleep, you should simply relax and rest your hold on the states of body and mind. If you enter into the death process in devotional heart-recognition of Me and heart-response to Me, resorting to Me to the point of utter self surrender, self-forgetting, and self-transcendence, then the event will suffer no distortion, and you will emerge into a right, profound, and ultimately happy destiny—even as such self-surrender, self-forgetting, and self-transcendence relieve your life, and sleep, and dreams of distortion, fear, illusion, and doubt while you live in this world.

And death is not a permanent event or effect. It is only a transition to further experience. It is a transforming event that prepares you for another birth, just as it stands before you, motivating you toward self-transcending surrender during your lifetime. Death and rebirth are the inevitable cycle of your existence, until you out-grow the limits of the conditional world, and Realize My Avatarically Self-Revealed (and Inherently Free, and Self-Evidently Divine) Self-Condition Most Perfectly.

So be it.

The Vision of Eternal Life

from *The Way That I Teach*

The great message of the universe is not that you survive. It is that you are awakened into a process in which nothing ultimately survives. Everything ultimately changes. Everything that rises also falls. Everything in its process of appearance is inevitably locked into a cycle that is changing. The Law you perceive in this life, then, is the Law of the obligation to be a sacrifice, to yield one's independent position. To hold on to one's position is a torment, producing all kinds of illusions and false hopes. It also makes you ego-possessed and loveless. Therefore, such clinging prevents your life, even while it continues, from becoming a creative form of participation and action.

As long as you are essentially ego-possessed and afraid, you look for consoling knowledge. You want to hear that you survive, you want to hear that there is something you can do in your room for twenty minutes each morning and evening that will make you Happy, because you do not want to go through the sacrifice, the <u>moral</u> change. You do not want to fulfill the Law. You do not want to lose face. You are always seeking to know in order to protect yourself. You want to save yourself and continue. And you cannot.

When you become aware of the message of things, and the Law of things, and the Truth of things, then you become combined with this affair of existence in an entirely different way. You see that the ultimate communication of the universe is Eternal Life. It is an Eternal Process. However, it is Eternal Life paradoxically expressed through a procession of infinite changes in which you are fundamentally without knowledge. If you can come into this certainty of Ignorance, you will feel profound relief. You will be already mindless, bodiless, beginningless, endless in your feeling, in your certainty, in your awareness itself—while at the same time paradoxically present in the mechanics of things. And through that Intuition you will become animated by the Law that obliges you, the Law of Sacrifice. You will fulfill the Law through love rather than pursue knowledge, certainty, and survival.

It is only when you are not certain of Ignorance that you pursue survival in the conventional sense, that you fail to make this sacrifice through love. Spiritual life is moral transformation through love, though feeling-Intuition of What <u>Is</u>. It is not a matter of gaining knowledge. All knowledge passes. There is no way to have any fixed certainty about whether or how you survive your death. You will never acquire any ultimate certainty through the means of knowledge. Yes—it is true that you are not smothered, ended, murdered. The universe is not a machine of death. But you will not become certain of Eternal Life through any egoic pursuit of certainty, knowledge, or information. All the forms of information ultimately contradict one another. You will realize that certainty only through devotional recognition-response to Me, through intelligent response to My Teaching Argument, through your commitment to the ego-surrendering, ego-forgetting, and (more and more) ego-transcending practice of Adidam, through love, through the energy of the whole body-being, through moment to moment devotional Communion with Me. You will enjoy a different Vision, not a vision realized through knowledge or egoic independence, but the Vision realized through the paradoxical disposition of the devotee: the Vision of Eternal Life, the Vision of Real God.

Only Life Overcomes Death

March 13, 1980

Death does not happen to Life. Only that which is merely touched and enlivened by Life can die (or seem to become Lifeless). But That Which is Alive is deathless and never threatened. The Self-Existing Being in Whom Man inheres Is Life. And Life is only conserved and increased by the process of changes or transformations. Life always persists, even after change and death.

Therefore, the idea that you are all going to die is simply false. It is a false, self-frustrating, and deluding presumption. "I" inheres in Life—and to believe otherwise is to embrace fear, separation, unlove, and all the philosophy that presumes death, rather than Life, to be the Principle of Existence. The idea that "I" can, will, or must die is a false belief, even a deadly act, founded on the failure to fully observe, "consider", and understand your experience. When true understanding arises, there is only the natural and positive presumption of Life, which inherently transcends experience, change, and death through the transforming power of Love-Surrender.

The Living Divine Being is not merely outside you and, thus, separate from your essential being. Nor is the Living Divine Being merely within you and, thus, separate from the body and the world. Rather, you wholly inhere in the Living Divine Being.

Therefore, the Way of Life is neither a matter of extroversion nor of introversion, but it is a matter of conversion, or ego-transcending heart-Communion with Me, the Infinitely Radiant and Eternally Living Divine Being. The Practice is feeling-surrender of body, mind, and attention—directly and via every kind of right or appropriate action—to the point or degree of Ecstasy, or Radiant Fullness of Life, beyond doubt and sorrow and fear.

Only Life overcomes death. Therefore, surrender to the Life-Principle and presume only Life to be your situation.

Original Light

from *Scientific Proof of the Existence of God Will Soon Be Announced by the White House!*

The conventions of sense experience habituate human beings to the idea that light is always generated from a defined source, specific locus, or point in space. It is this presumption that permits human beings to perceive and conceive of defined or differentiated objects, space between objects, relative degrees of illumination, and also shadows. But, truly, all space, all locations, all objects are equally Pervaded by Indivisible Light, Universal Energy, or Transcendental, Inherently Spiritual, and Self-Evidently Divine Self-Radiance. If you "consider" the nature of perception and cognition within that Light, which is omnidirectional or Infinite, then you realize that not objects, no degrees of light, no shadows, no differences can be found therein. Just so, if you Realize Ecstasy, or perfect inherence in the Indivisible Light wherein all objects or conventions of difference appear, then you transcend all differences, all states of body, mind, space, time, "self", and relations.

True Ecstasy in the Living Divine Reality is self-transcending inherence in the selfless, mindless, bodiless, worldless Infinity of Self-Existing and Self-Radiant Love-Bliss-Happiness. Real God, Truth, or Reality Itself That is only Obvious and not to be identified with any independently subjective or objective states, Is Infinite Light, the condition of all conditions or permutations of light-energy. You must enter into the Presumption of That Condition via your native transcending of the conventions of psycho-physical experience. Then that same Light will transform you in every part, until there is not the slightest difference between you and that uninterrupted Divine Glory.

My Sphere of Love-Bliss

Epilogue from *Ishta*

AVATAR ADI DA SAMRAJ: The Work I Do is at the Source-Point, without "difference". The Work I Do does not require any cosmic designs, or any visualizations, or any traveling to support it.

I Am at the Source.

I Am the Source Itself.

By merely Being, I Do My Work. Not via conditions, not supported by conditions at all.

The Power of Being Itself is the Intimate Beyond Intimate Space of Absolute Delight. Without complication. No subject and object.

Real God Is Source. Beyond conditions, Beyond visualizations, Beyond objects.

Real God Is Love-Bliss, Unsupported, Free.

You are full of fear. Yet you possess psychological mechanisms with which you immunize yourself against your fundamental fear.

You experience fear as just a kind of stress or anxiety, a motivation to seek. Yet you are actually looking into the face of that terrible deity of your infinitely magnified separateness.

Rather than looking for the source of your fear, you must transcend fear through heart-Communion with Me.

Give yourself up to Me.

Give yourself up to the Divine, truly.

Surrender yourself.

Forget yourself.

That process is full of My Love-Bliss and magnifies only My Love-Bliss, not fear.

Your reluctance to practice Ruchira Avatara Bhakti is a movement toward your fear.

The real practice of Ruchira Avatara Bhakti always reveals more and more Freedom, more and more Love-Bliss, more and more heart-Communion with the God Who truly Is, not the mere "maker" of events but the Divine Who Transcends all, Who Is All Love-Bliss, Who Is utterly Free, Who Is not contained, not confined, not supported by conditions.

The True Divine is utterly without fear, and does not cause fear in any experience of It.

Your heart-Communion with Me does not cause fear to arise.

Notice this.

If you truly practice Ruchira Avatara Bhakti Yoga, if you truly practice heart-Communion with Me, your fear is weakened and purified.

The moments of real heart-Communion with Me have no fear in them. They do not magnify fear.

Notice this.

This is how you grasp at heart, more profoundly, that the Way of Adidam is Truth, because it does not magnify fear.

If you practice the Way of Adidam even a little bit, there is that much less fear.

The sign of your true practice of Ruchira Avatara Bhakti Yoga, your true heart-Communion with Me, shows itself as weakening of fear, and this sign inspires you further.

When you surrender to Me, your fear is weakened and dissolved, so that you go further, surrender more, forget yourself more.

The worst thing of all is the fear. It is the primal sign of the self-contraction, the root-sign of egoity.

The more you practice devotion to Me, the less you experience fear, but also the less you experience anxiety.

The knot of self-contraction is dissolved, washed through, such that there is less and less of it and more and more of the profound investment in My Love-Bliss.

This is the Way of Adidam, the Way of the Yoga of devotion to Me.

All seeking, all clinging to objectivity, all clinging to objects of any kind, intensifies first your anxiety and then your fear.

Fear is the first artifact of your egoity. It is behind everything you do.

Practice devotion to Me moment by moment, and there is less and less of anxiety, less and less of fear, more and more fullness of Love-Bliss.

Do you not notice this?

The process of self-surrender and self-forgetting relinquishes the point of view of the body-mind.

This is how you go beyond the potential of the dark vision, beyond your fear, and beyond your anxiety also.

You fear the absence of objective signs.

You fear the absence of the "difference" that your body makes and your mind makes.

Yet these are exactly the categories of existence you must go beyond in your surrender to Me.

The Ultimate Delight is bodiless, and mindless.

That is the Freedom.

That is the Realization.

It is also the Context of any Work I may Do beyond the Lifetime of This Body—if there is any Work left over for Me to Do.

For My devotee, the seventh stage Realization is bodiless, and mindless.

The body-mind is not the point of view of the seventh stage Realization.

Likewise, the body-mind is not the point of view of heart-Communion with Me.

The body-mind is the point of view that is the source of fear.

Therefore, you are afraid of death.

And, afraid of death, you are afraid of the very Process That is your Freedom!

That Process is a profoundly, ultimately Most Perfectly, Subjective Process—not an historical event whereby the cosmic domain disappears, as if in opposition to the "big bang" that supposedly made it happen to begin with.

Your heart-Communion with Me is beyond the separate self—therefore, beyond the body-mind.

By your persistence in Ruchira Avatara Bhakti Yoga, you will transcend your fear.

Even so, if such transcending is to occur, the point of view of the body-mind must be relinquished in heart-Communion with Me.

The body-mind is what there is to forget.

The self-contraction, yes, but also the context and structure of the self-contraction.

Relinquish this point of view.

There is mere physical death.

But I am Talking about something greater—the true Process of ego-surrendering and ego-forgetting that transcends the point of view of the body-mind.

That is the death I am Talking about.

That death is the import of true religion.

That death is not a suicide, not a struggle with the body.

That death is heart-Communion with the Very Divine to the degree that you forget the body-mind rather than struggle with it.

The body-mind must cease to be your point of view, not merely cease to exist.

If you practice this Yoga of devotion to Me, then the point of view of the body-mind—and, therefore, all the reflection of self-contraction, all the fear—is surrendered and forgotten, dissolved in that surrendering and forgetting.

This is how you will unlearn your fear of death.

Natural death is just a natural phenomenon.

What you fear about it is the fear associated with your self-contraction, or the point of view of your body-mind.

You enter into My Sphere of Love-Bliss by transcending that point of view through Ruchira Avatara Bhakti Yoga, so that all of your anxiety about natural death and the potential suffering in life likewise vanishes.

The event itself, death itself, occurs in any case. It is a natural phenomenon.

You must be in My Sphere.

In that heart-Communion with Me, your anxieties are released, and your fear.

Then another destiny becomes yours—just by this surrender, this forgetting, this heart-Communion with Me, this participation in Me, this transition into My Sphere.

My Divine Translation, this Bhava, is My Experience all the time.

Yet My apparent Association with you, and with this conditional domain, Continues without bondage.

Ultimately, My Divine Translation is simply the Relinquishment of My Active Gestures within the cosmic domain.

My Divine Translation is not the end of My Gestures altogether, not the end of My Work, not the end of My Influence.

My Standing Firm in the Divine Domain is My Greatest Attractiveness, My Greatest Influence, My Greatest Siddhi, and It is already Happening.

Still, I Remain Influential within this conditional sphere, Mysteriously—just long enough that I am Satisfied. Or, better said, just long enough that I Forget it.

I Am not truly here on the basis of concerns.

I animate apparent concerns for your sake.

My Certainty is that My Siddhi of Divine Translation is the Ultimate Means whereby My Work will be Effective throughout the cosmic domain, forever.

Do the sadhana I have Given you to do with all your responsibilities, and leave Me in My Samadhi, Shining here and everywhere.

Let that be the basis of your relationship to Me.

You are in a fluid position with Me—always moving on.

Therefore, address My Leela, and keep moving with Me.

Fulfill your responsibilities, do your practice, and always enter into ego-surrendering and ego-forgetting heart-Communion with Me.

Keep moving with Me.

I am Moving constantly—and Moveless, also.

All My Movements are mere appearances in the Place of My Standing Firm.

When you truly come to Me, the rooms, the movements, and the places will disintegrate and you will Wake Up to Where you Have always Been, Where you always already Are.

All the appearances of movement are a play, an illusion, within which you must do sadhana.

Resort to Me and understand yourself.

Do not take anything that is conditional seriously.

Take Me seriously.

Practice Ruchira Avatara Bhakti Yoga, surrendering and forgetting your self-position, all your faculties, all apparent relations, all seemings—with nothing to hold onto but Me.

If you think life is difficult, watch death!

Death is a profound intrusion as a merely natural event.

My devotees, Communing with Me most profoundly, must be released of all the horrors of the suffering of life, and also of death.

Yet you are rather casual about life and death, because you can enjoy your social congeniality, your social consolation, your functional consolation. You can just keep it orderly, keep the consolations going.

In heart-Communion with Me, even your intimacies are about surrender—not the consolation, not the holding on, not the congeniality of this appearance here that is presumed to be eternal.

Intimate relations, if they exist, even friendships, must be a circumstance of your devotion to Me, your surrender—not your holding on, not your consolation.

This apparent order is a moment made by your fear.

None of it will continue.

It is a while that tests you, that tests the choice you will make—to hold on to it or to surrender.

Nobody is going to go with you to the whirring place at death, where mind makes existence.

Nor is anyone with you now—but Me.

Yet, on the basis of the point of view of the body-mind, you assume relations, and the apparent order, and the would-be consolations.

You are holding on instead of surrendering.

You are creating an idol, an alternative to the Divine, made of your consolations, your arrangements, your attempts to fill the anxiety and somehow forget it.

The darkness of ego-possessed mind after death is a whirring terror.

It is not fun.

Nor are you having fun now!

You are not having any fun at all.

You are just deluding yourself to reduce your anxiety.

All your arrangements and consolations are just efforts on your part to reduce your anxiety.

Yet you are right in the face of this terrible place of your confinement and separateness.

You must become serious in My Company—serious about the reality in which you are existing and which is making you fear it.

You are full of fear and anxiety.

Fear and anxiety make you seek and make consolations and arrangements, as if your consolations will go on forever.

You must appreciate the game you are playing.

You must understand that it is based on fear.

You must respond to Me and transform every aspect of your life through self-surrender and self-forgetting, making all of life a Yoga, rather than an indulgence in things that console you.

People who indulge themselves in consolations are not serious.

I cannot take them seriously, and I cannot trust them.

Therefore, do this Yoga.

Keep on growing.

Get closer and closer to Me.

Be serious.

Stay in My Company.

Do not let up for a moment.

If you are intelligent, you would not dare let up for a moment.

Therefore, become more intelligent.

Stay with Me, and you can afford to be quiet.

Do you ever get quiet—just quiet?

Talking the cool blueness, the full moonlit night, consciousness attendant to the Divine, all energy flowing, even running out of the top of the head like a fountain.

Undisturbed.

Not seeking.

Invested utterly in Me.

That is it.

Not stimulations and consolations.

You are not in a paradise of Western democracy.

You are in a terrible night of fear.

You keep agitating yourself toward consolations, so that you will not have to experience your state—which is superficially anxious and deeply afraid.

What you would have in heart-Communion with Me is a cool, watery, full moonlit night, cooled of stress, and desire, and consolation, Awake to "Brightness".

On that basis, visions of clarity and peace.

And then moving beyond them to My Love-Bliss Itself, without the slightest image, without the slightest object, without the slightest fear, without any "other"—not even yourself an "other".

No "other".
No separation.
No visions.
No objects.

Only Self-Existing Being, Self-Radiant without limitation.

No separate self.
No objects.
No cosmos.
No seeking.

Samadhi.
Samadana.
Utterly rested.
Fearless.
Unmoved.

No place.
No going and coming.
No conversation.
No society.
No world.
No sex organs.
No thing.
But Fullness Itself, not objective.

Only Real God.
Only "Brightness".
No "difference".
No relatedness.
Only Happiness.
No un-Happiness.
No threat.

This is What there is to be Realized, not the mayhem you are manufacturing in your fear and seeking, in your contraction into separateness.

Devote your life to this Peace Beyond "difference", this Divinity, this heart-Communion with Me.

Everything else is just something to be noticed, just a discipline to be applied, more intense practice of this devotion to Me.

All the superficial matter temporary, not important.

Be still.
Be washed.

Be mindless.
Bodiless.
Sublime.
Real God Only.

"We are Home now, Lord."

That is it.
Do not leave.

PART SEVEN

Legal Documents

Directions for Completing the Durable Power of Attorney for Health Care

Following is a copy of the Durable Power of Attorney for Health Care (DPAHC) which is legal in the state of California (with extra wording about our religious beliefs). If you wish to have a non-devotee complete a DPAHC, do not use this one, but obtain a form from an attorney, hospital, or hospice organization in your geographic area. If you do not live in California, you should use a form which is legal where you live. The wording pertaining to your wishes and instructions as a practitioner of Adidam (including instructions about disposition of the body after death) which are contained in the California DPAHC at the back of this guide should be added to your DPAHC in consultation with an appropriate legal professional in your jurisdiction. Be sure your DPAHC (or its equivalent in your jurisdiction) allows you to name people to make health care decisions for you if you are unable to do so (a living will generally does not do this).

After filling out the DPAHC, make a copy to give to your Mate Moce or Clinic representative and keep the original yourself. Yellow alert cards will be available in each region from your CSM or Mate Moce representative. Keep the card with you at all times, preferably next to your driver's license, letting anyone know, in case of emergency, who to call.

In the DPAHC use your legal name, the name you would use if you were to go to a hospital. Use black ink so copies will be clear.

If you are a resident of California, the DPAHC at the back of this guide meets the legal requirements in California for this document at the time of publication of this manual. Print your name on page 1. In section IV print your name, then fill in your representatives (or attorneys-in-fact). The first name is generally your spouse or your intimate partner or a family member who is a practitioner of Adidam. This should be followed by two close friends or family members in your regional Adidam community. It is best to use the names of other Adidam members over non-devotee family or friends, because members of Adidam would be willing to follow the instructions Beloved Adi Da has Given us as they pertain to the matter of death and dying. Talk with those you list on your DPAHC. It is a big responsibility. Another note about choosing these people. The representative you name does not need to be the person you would most want to provide emotional support at time of death. This person needs to be one who can deal effectively with authority figures and can make clear decisions (presumably with help from other members of the culture and Radiant Life Clinic).

In section VI (9) it says, "I request that my body be cremated, and the ashes scattered —" You may leave this blank or state where you want your ashes scattered. Beloved Adi Da has Told us not to scatter ashes on or near Sanctuaries.

After section VIII there is a place for signing and witnessing. Sign in the presence of both your witnesses. Read out loud and to your witnesses carefully the section regarding the witnesses' declarations. Please note your witnesses will print their name, write their signature, the date and their residential address after the first witness declaration entitled "Statement of Witness". There is a further declaration on the final page of the DPAHC which again requires the signatures of both witnesses. Witnesses may not be one of the people you have named in the DPAHC, or your health care provider or a family member. With two witnesses signing this document, it does not have to be notarized, but doing so would add to its clout.

DO NOT COMPLETE THIS FORM WITHOUT CAREFULLY READING THE COMPLETE INSTRUCTIONS CONTAINED IN THE "DIRECTIONS FOR COMPLETING THE DURABLE POWER OF ATTORNEY FOR HEALTH CARE" ON PAGE 112.

Durable Power of Attorney for Health Care

My name is ____.

I. WARNING TO PERSON EXECUTING THIS DOCUMENT

THIS IS AN IMPORTANT LEGAL DOCUMENT. BEFORE EXECUTING THIS DOCUMENT, YOU SHOULD KNOW THESE IMPORTANT FACTS:

THIS DOCUMENT GIVES THE PERSON YOU DESIGNATE AS YOUR AGENT (THE ATTORNEY-IN-FACT) THE POWER TO MAKE HEALTH CARE DECISIONS FOR YOU. YOUR AGENT MUST ACT CONSISTENTLY WITH YOUR DESIRES AS STATED IN THIS DOCUMENT OR OTHERWISE MADE KNOWN.

EXCEPT AS YOU OTHERWISE SPECIFY IN THIS DOCUMENT, THIS DOCUMENT GIVES YOUR AGENT THE POWER TO CONSENT TO YOUR DOCTOR NOT GIVING TREATMENT OR STOPPING TREATMENT NECESSARY TO KEEP YOU ALIVE.

NOTWITHSTANDING THIS DOCUMENT, YOU HAVE THE RIGHT TO MAKE MEDICAL AND OTHER HEALTH CARE DECISIONS FOR YOURSELF SO LONG AS YOU CAN GIVE INFORMED CONSENT WITH RESPECT TO THE PARTICULAR DECISION. IN ADDITION, NO TREATMENT MAY BE GIVEN TO YOU OVER YOUR OBJECTION AT THE TIME, AND HEALTH CARE NECESSARY TO KEEP YOU ALIVE MAY NOT BE STOPPED OR WITHHELD IF YOU OBJECT AT THE TIME.

THIS DOCUMENT GIVES YOUR AGENT AUTHORITY TO CONSENT, TO REFUSE TO CONSENT, OR TO WITHDRAW CONSENT TO ANY CARE, TREATMENT, SERVICE, OR PROCEDURE TO MAINTAIN, DIAGNOSE, OR TREAT A PHYSICAL OR MENTAL CONDITION. THIS POWER IS SUBJECT TO ANY STATEMENT OF YOUR DESIRES AND ANY LIMITATIONS THAT YOU INCLUDE IN THIS DOCUMENT. YOU MAY STATE IN THIS DOCUMENT ANY TYPES OF TREATMENT THAT YOU DO NOT DESIRE. IN ADDITION, A COURT CAN TAKE AWAY THE POWER OF YOUR AGENT TO MAKE HEALTH CARE DECISIONS FOR YOU IF YOUR AGENT (1) AUTHORIZES ANYTHING THAT IS ILLEGAL, (2) ACTS CONTRARY TO YOUR KNOWN DESIRES, OR (3) WHERE YOUR DESIRES ARE NOT KNOWN, DOES ANYTHING THAT IS CLEARLY CONTRARY TO YOUR BEST INTERESTS.

THIS POWER WILL EXIST FOR AN INDEFINITE PERIOD OF TIME UNLESS YOU LIMIT ITS DURATION IN THIS DOCUMENT.

YOU HAVE THE RIGHT TO REVOKE THE AUTHORITY OF YOUR AGENT BY NOTIFYING YOUR AGENT OR YOUR TREATING DOCTOR, HOSPITAL, OR OTHER HEALTH CARE PROVIDER ORALLY OR IN WRITING OF THE REVOCATION.

YOUR AGENT HAS THE RIGHT TO EXAMINE YOUR MEDICAL RECORDS AND TO CONSENT TO THEIR DISCLOSURE UNLESS YOU LIMIT THIS RIGHT IN THIS DOCUMENT.

UNLESS YOU OTHERWISE SPECIFY IN THIS DOCUMENT, THIS DOCUMENT GIVES YOUR AGENT THE POWER AFTER YOU DIE TO (1) AUTHORIZE AN AUTOPSY, (2) DONATE YOUR BODY OR PARTS THEREOF FOR TRANSPLANT OR THERAPEUTIC OR EDUCATIONAL OR SCIENTIFIC PURPOSES, AND (3) DIRECT THE DISPOSITION OF YOUR REMAINS.

IF THERE IS ANYTHING IN THIS DOCUMENT THAT YOU DO NOT UNDERSTAND, YOU SHOULD ASK A LAWYER TO EXPLAIN IT TO YOU.

II. Creation and Duration of Durable Power of Attorney for Health Care

By this document I intend to create a Durable Power of Attorney for Health Care as authorized by the California Probate Code. This power of attorney shall remain in force despite my subsequent incapacity. This power of attorney is effective immediately and shall remain in force indefinitely.

III. Statement of Intent of Creation of This Document

I have strong personal and religious beliefs about the type of health care I should receive if, due to serious illness or injury, I were to become incompetent and incapable of determining my own health care future. Therefore, I want to make it clear to all my treating health care practitioners, the health care agent(s) I designate in this document, and everyone else (including any judge or state official) what my feeling are regarding the medical treatment I should receive if I become unable to make my own health care decisions. My church is Adidam, and this document reflects my personal and religious beliefs; if you are unclear or have questions about my beliefs, please consult my regional minister of Adidam.

I expressly intend that this document be given full legal force and effect in whatever country or jurisdiction I may be in. Accordingly, failure to follow my health care directions, or those of my acting health care agent(s) designated herein, would violate my human rights and be an affront to my personal dignity.

My intent in this document is to create a Durable Power of Attorney for Health Care decisions as allowed by the laws of the state of California. The person(s) I name in this document as my health care agent (also known as my Attorney-in-fact) is authorized to make health care decisions for me if I am incapacitated. This health care power of attorney shall continue even if I am incapacitated in the future.

IV. Appointment of Health Care Agent (Attorney-in-Fact)

I, ____, appoint the following persons in the order listed to be my health care agent to make health care decisions for me as authorized in and consistent with this document. I always have the power and right to substitute another attorney-in-fact or to revoke this appointment.

1. ________________________________;

2. ________________________________;

3. ________________________________.

When I appoint persons in numerical order, it is my intention that the person(s) named first be the first to serve as my health care agent, and if that person(s) for any reason does not serve, then the next person(s) shall serve. I request that all persons listed above be notified in event that this document becomes effective and my health care agent is acting.

V. Statement on Authority Granted to Health Care Agent

In paragraph VI below I state specific authority given to my health care agent. In addition, however, if I become unable to give informed consent for health care decisions, I grant to my health care agent full power and authority to make health care decisions for me consistent with my beliefs and directions as stated in this document. This authority includes, but is not limited to, the following: right to give or refuse consent, or withdraw consent to any care, treatment, service, or procedure, to maintain, diagnose, or treat a physical or mental condition, and the right to ask for and receive medical information, or consent to the release of medical information, the right to obtain, retain, or discharge any health care practitioner or health care facility.

I also give my health care agent the right to make funeral arrangements, sign cremation permits and transfer, transport, and make any arrangements for my body after death which my health care agent deems necessary or consistent in his/her sole judgement with my wishes as expressed in this document.

Further, I give my health care agent full authority to use all reasonable means, including legal action, to carry out my directions as expressed in this document and to exercise the specific authority granted him/her herein.

VI. Delegation of Powers

(1) My attorney-in-fact, as designated in this document, has priority over all other persons to act on my behalf in all matters relating to my health care, unless I am able to give informed consent with respect to such matters.

(2) The person(s) I designate in this document may make health care decisions for me, before or after my death, to the same extent I could. However, this power specifically does not include making any disposition(s) under the Uniform Anatomical Gift Act. The person(s) designated herein must act consistent with my wishes if expressed, or, if unknown, in my best interest.

(3) I hereby declare that, despite my desire to live and enjoy life as long as possible, I nevertheless do not wish to prolong my life at all costs. I believe that life is part of a greater process that includes life and death, and what is beyond death. I believe death is not a final event, but a necessary and ultimately benign psycho-physical event. Accordingly, I express my wish that my life not be prolonged by artificial means (including but not limited to respirators and intravenous feeding, nasogastric tube, gastrostomy, or cardiopulmonary resuscitation) and that I be permitted to die in peace, free of active medical intervention, if:

(a) I have undergone an irreversible cessation of total spontaneous brain function; or

(b) I have a terminal, irreversible condition, or there is no reasonable medical expectation of recovery whether I am conscious or not; or

(c) The following statement of my general desires is met: I do not want my life to be prolonged, and I do not want life sustaining treatment to be provided or continued, if the burdens of the treatment to be provided or continued, outweigh the expected benefits. I want my agent to consider the relief of suffering and the quality of my life, as well as the extent of the possible extension of my life, in making decisions concerning life-sustaining treatment; or

(d) If I am a woman, terminally ill or seriously injured, and I am pregnant, I ask that every reasonable medical treatment be given to bring my baby to term, including, for example, keeping me alive while I am "brain dead" or in an irreversible coma. I also ask, however, that after the baby is born, or if it dies while in my womb, that all life support then be withdrawn after notifying my health care agent and church representatives.

If my attorney-in-fact determines that any of the above situations exists, I authorize him/her to discontinue the use of some or all of any medication being given to me, or the use of life-sustaining devices upon which I am dependent. I give my agent broad discretionary powers to make medical decisions on my behalf.

If I am terminally ill or seriously injured and not able to consciously determine my own health care needs nor communicate coherently and interact with others, I ask and direct that health care givers (medical staff, etc.), as well as my intimates, relatives and friends, accept the direction of my health care agent as to my wishes for my health care and future. I also ask and direct that health care givers, intimates, relatives and friends respect and allow, without obstruction or impedance, the acts or rituals that my church representatives offer to or perform for me during the death process.

(4) Whether I am terminally ill or not, if I am unable to make medical decisions for myself, my attorney-in-fact is hereby authorized to use his/her best judgment in determining what medications, if any, I should take, and what operations, if any, I should undergo.

Although I wish to consciously participate in my death, I ask that medication be mercifully administered to me to alleviate suffering and control pain. I am aware that such medication may shorten my life.

(5) I desire that my wishes in this regard be carried out, despite the contrary feelings, beliefs or opinions of my immediate family, other relatives or friends, and

(6) When I die, I ask and direct that my body not be autopsied nor organs removed for study or donation.

(7) During the first two to three hours after the cessation of all vital signs in the body, I want to be left undisturbed except for those services which are deemed necessary by those I have designated to serve my death transition, being my church representatives, in coordination with my health care agent.

(8) If my death is imminent, if at all possible I desire to die in a private home or Sanctuary environment, surrounded and served by my church representatives and understanding friends, and to be left undisturbed therein for a period of two to three days, until my church representatives have determined that my body is ready for cremation.

(9) I request that my body be cremated, and the ashes scattered as follows:

____

____

____.

VII. Reliance on Photocopies

Any person dealing with my health care agent shall have the right to rely on a photocopy of this Durable Power of Attorney for Health Care, certified by my health care agent as being genuine, as if it were the signed, original Durable Power of Attorney for Health Care.

VIII. Nomination of Conservator

If a court finds it necessary to appoint a conservator of my person then I nominate the person(s) named under Article IV of this document, as listed there, to serve as such conservator without bond.

SIGNING:

I, ______________________________________, have carefully read this document. I understand completely the significance of this document, including the significance of all of the powers I grant herein to my attorney-in-fact for health care. Acting on the basis of that understanding, I hereby sign this Durable Power of Attorney on the date shown below my signature, intending thereby that this document have full legal effect in accordance with its terms. I understand (1) this document gives my attorney-in-fact (health care agent) serious powers over me; (2) the powers continue after I am disabled; and (3) I can revoke and cancel this document at any time.

____

PRINTED NAME

____

SIGNATURE

____

DATE

Executed in the City of ____________________________________, State of California.

STATEMENT OF WITNESS:

I declare under penalty of perjury under the laws of California that the person who signed or acknowledged this instrument is personally known to me to be the principal, or that the identity of the principal was proved to me by convincing evidence, that the principal signed or acknowledged this Durable Power of Attorney for Health Care in my presence, that the principal appears to be of sound mind and under no duress, fraud, or undue influence, that I am not the person appointed as attorney-in-fact by this document, and that I am not the principal's health care provider, an employee of the principal's health care provider, the operator of a community care facility, an employee of an operator of a community care facility, the operator of a residential care facility for the elderly, nor an employee of the operator of a residential care facility for the elderly.

WITNESS ONE:

____

PRINTED NAME

____

SIGNATURE

____

DATE

____

RESIDENTIAL ADDRESS

WITNESS TWO:

____

PRINTED NAME

____

SIGNATURE

____

DATE

____

RESIDENTIAL ADDRESS

I further declare under penalty of perjury under the laws of California, that I am not related to the principal by blood, marriage, or adoption, and, to the best of my knowledge, I am not entitled to any part of the estate of the principal upon the death of the principal under a will now existing or by operation of law.

____

SIGNATURE

____

SIGNATURE

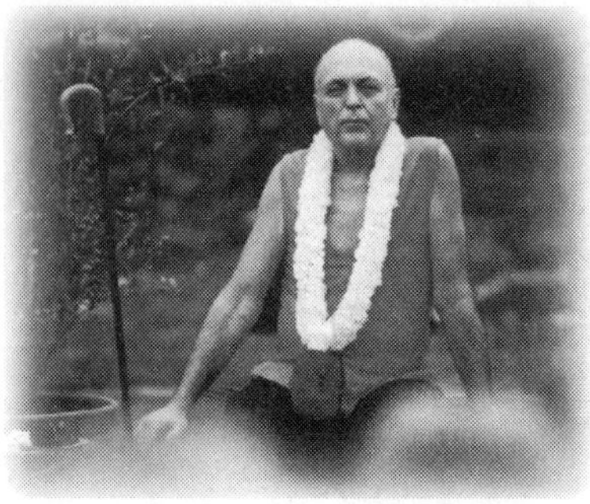

How You Can Respond To Avatar Adi Da Samraj

■ **Contact us to sign up for one of our classes, correspondence courses, seminars, events, or retreats—or to find the regional center nearest you.**

AMERICAS
12040 N. Seigler Rd.
Middletown, CA
95461 USA
(707) 928-4936

PACIFIC-ASIA
12 Seibel Road
Henderson
Auckland 1008
New Zealand
64-9-838-9114

AUSTRALIA
P.O. Box 460
Roseville,
NSW 2069
Australia
61-2-9419-7563

EUROPE-AFRICA
Annendaalderweg 10
6105 AT Maria Hoop
The Netherlands
31 (0)20 468 1442

THE UNITED KINGDOM
P.O. Box 20013
London, England
NW2 1ZA
0181-7317550

E-MAIL: correspondence@adidam.org

■ **Order more books by and about Avatar Adi Da Samraj**.
(877) 770-0772 (from within North America)
(707) 928-6653 (from outside North America)
order on-line: http://www.adidam.com

■ **Visit the Adidam website: http://www.adidam.org**
- See photographs of Avatar Adi Da Samraj.
- Hear audio-clips of Him Speaking.
- Read His Writings and Stories of His Divine Work.
- Find a complete listing of all our regional centers and mission groups worldwide.